THE PURSUIT OF HEALTH

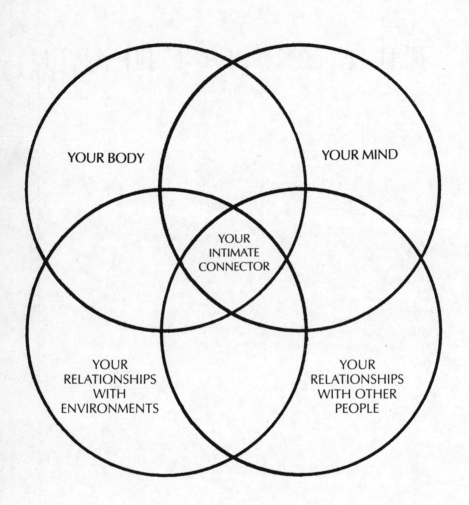

YOUR BODY

YOUR MIND

YOUR INTIMATE CONNECTOR

YOUR RELATIONSHIPS WITH ENVIRONMENTS

YOUR RELATIONSHIPS WITH OTHER PEOPLE

THE PURSUIT OF HEALTH

June Bingham and
Norman Tamarkin, M.D.

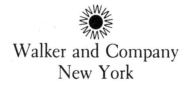

Walker and Company
New York

First published in the United States of America
in 1985 by the Walker Publishing Company, Inc.

Published simultaneously in Canada by John Wiley & Sons
Canada, Limited, Rexdale, Ontario

Library of Congress Cataloging in Publication Data

Bingham, June, 1919–
  Pursuit of health.

  Includes index.
  1. Holistic medicine. 2. Medicine, Psychosomatic.
3. Mind and body. 4. Health. I. Tamarkin, Norman.
II. Title.
R733.B56 1985   616.89'05   85-10595
ISBN 0-8027-0869-2

Printed in the United States of America

10 9 8 7 6 5 4 3 2 1

To the memory of Dr. Rudolph Kaelbling

and to the good health of the following wise questioners:
Jonathan B. Bingham
Micki B. Esselstyn
Mary Z. Gray, and
Richard K. Winslow, our editor.

Contents

For a physician and a writer to collaborate on a book has one advantage. Their lines of responsibility remain clear. When the question concerns medical fact or interpretation, the doctor has the last word. When the question concerns whether, or how, to include this fact or interpretation, the writer has the last word.

These authors, nonetheless, discovered other problems. One was the vastness of their self-assigned subject: to devise a conceptual model for *all* of health. Although the book itself cannot encompass every form of well-being and disease, theoretically, the model should be able to.

The second problem concerned the authors' own health during the five years of weekly health discussions. First the writer had to have a spinal disc taken out; then the physician had to have a heart valve put in. This, friends told them, was carrying their research too far!

Yet today, touch wood, both authors are back on the tennis court, thanks in large measure to their reminding each other to apply in daily life the book's underlying concept. In short, it works!

I
The Dimensions of Health

*"Contentment preserves one even from catching cold.
Has a woman who knew she was well dressed ever
caught cold?—No, not even when she had scarcely
a rag to her back."*

—Nietzsche

Today's mind-body (psycho-somatic) approach to health is not as new as some people assume. King Solomon, for one, was explicit on the subject: "A merry heart doeth good like medicine, but a broken spirit drieth the bone."

The obverse, the body-mind (somato-psychic) approach is even older. The first cavewoman who sampled a button-shaped mushroom doubtless sang her way back to that glade, followed, in time, by the rest of the band. As with peyote, so with fermented grape juice.

What is new is that today's tools are refined enough to track some of the millions of complex brain events that link the body with the mind, and both with the world outside. For example, my joy in seeing you, a *subjective* feeling, can now be *objectively* spotted through measurable changes in my brain waves and blood chemistry. These, in turn, are connected with the subtle flow—or ebb—of neurochemicals and electrical impulses in my brain.

My health problems may thus be "all in my head," but in a biochemical or electromagnetic sense, rather than a purely psychological one. Yet even the most accurate sleuthing of mind-body interactions cannot always reveal why one person gets sick while another does not, or why someone gets sick today but does not tomorrow. Each individual's "health equation" needs, therefore, to be expanded beyond the psychosomatic and somatopsychic to include two further dimensions.

The first of these became evident in the latter half of the nineteenth century, when a Viennese neurologist focused on ways in which his patients' bodies and minds were affected by their relationship to *other people*. Even after such influential people were dead, their impact on the patient could remain potent enough to keep him paralyzed (body) or haunted by anxiety (mind).

Today, not all of Sigmund Freud's theories are endorsed by all psychiatrists—or even all psychoanalysts.* Yet few question the basic hypothesis, formulated by him and Drs. Jean Charcot and Josef Breuer, that thoroughly unconscious (repressed) interactions with other people can long influence not only our health of mind and body but also our behavior. A recent study by Anthony Marcel, a psychologist at the Medical Research Council in Cambridge, England, indicates that Freud *under*estimated the effect of the unconscious.

The second of these new dimensions became evident in the latter half of the twentieth century, when use of computers first alerted investigators to the impact on human well-being of previously unsuspected *environmental* factors. These include not only variations of light and sound, air and water, but also the values of the society in which the individual's life is embedded.

Our health's four dimensions are, therefore:

1. body
2. mind
3. relationship to other people
4. relationship to environments (physical and cultural)

And these dimensions never cease interacting with each other. Similarly, there is no rest for the inner force or process that keeps integrating them. When this core, or essence, of the person is in full operation, he feels "together," "centered," able to "cope"; when it is not, he feels as if he's "falling apart," "going to pieces," "coming apart at the seams." (See Fig. 1.)

This force or process often moves further into one of the four dimensions, but without losing touch with the others. In the athlete, for example, it moves primarily into body; in the professor, into mind; in the hostess, into relationships with people; in the explorer, into relationship with environments.

The central integrating force includes what some people call *spirit*,

*In simple terms, a *psychiatrist* must have an M.D., while a *psychoanalyst* must undergo an extensive training analysis. A licensed *psychotherapist* is likely to have been trained as a clinical psychologist or have earned an advanced degree in social work, education, or nursing.

Fig. 1

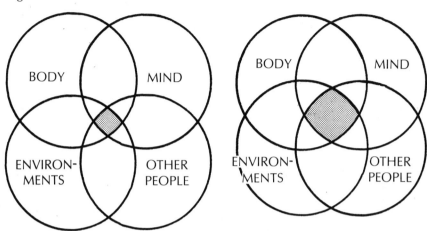

The person feels as if he's "falling apart."

The person feels "together."

what others call *soul*. It embraces both the will to live and the will to health (at times these two may be different). It also incorporates our capacity to surrender our life or health, for reasons either altruistic or selfish. The authors tried out and discarded some fifty names for this force before settling on the *intimate connector*. Yet even that name is not ideal, for the connector is also a connect*edness*. Still, the term *intimate connector* seemed a serendipitous one, in that it creates the acronym IC, or "I see!"

In daily terms, the IC is what people mean when they say "I."

"Here I stand," said Martin Luther. "I can do no other." And Thomas More, in Robert Bolt's *A Man for All Seasons*, was even more specific: "I will not give in because I oppose it—I do—not my pride, not my spleen, nor any other of my appetites, but I do. I."

Dr. Hans Zinsser, after a long life as a distinguished physican, wrote in his autobiography, "Here I am, my mind more alive and vivid than ever before . . . my affection stronger. . . . Yet here am I . . . held in a damaged body which will extinguish me when it dies. . . . No, no, my organs! I cannot feel that you have let me down. . . . Only now it

Fig. 2

The Intimate Connector
is constantly changing in *direction*.

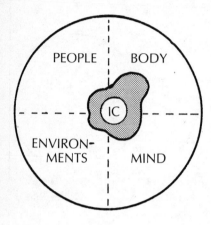

In the athlete, for example, the IC moves way over into *body*.

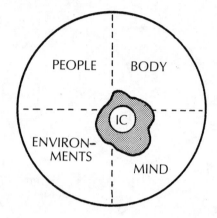

In the professor, the IC moves way over into *mind*.

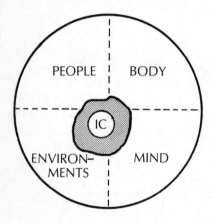

In the explorer, the IC moves way over into relationships with *environments*.

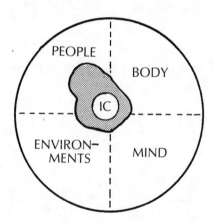

In the hostess, the IC moves way over into relationships with *people*.

feels so silly that you must take me with you when I am just beginning to get dry behind the ears."*

The human "I" is anything but a simple unit. It includes an acting self that is under surveillance by an observing self, which itself can be observed. The human is defined as the only creature that thinks about what it thinks about. Says a formerly ill schizophrenic, "All those years I was in the hospital, there was some part of me that knew I was acting crazy." And some criminally insane murderers, before fleeing the gruesome results of their crime, leave a note, in effect begging the police to catch them and thus prevent them from repeating the harm that one part of them was deploring while another part felt compelled to perpetrate it.

One wholesome example of how the IC expands the self's perspective on itself is that of a forty-five-year-old woman who, because of cancer, had to have both breasts removed. A nurse came into her hospital room a few nights after surgery and found her weeping.

"What's the problem?"

"I miss them."

"Listen. I saw you before the operation. You had beauties. And you had them for thirty years. Look at me. I've got nothing. And never will."

The patient looked at the nurse's flat chest—and then at her eyes, which combined human kindness with a professional no-nonsense quality. The miasma of depression in which she had been enveloped was pierced by a flash of objectivity. "No use crying over spilled milk, is there?" The nurse, startled, grinned. With each aware of the need to adjust to her own imperfection, both felt consoled.

The IC, furthermore, is the locus of the will, described by poet May Sarton as "the driver, the implacable *wanter* and *demander*." At the same time, the IC is also the locus of the capacity to surrender one's will.

Sometimes this surrender is involuntary, perhaps to a specific dimension of the self, as with addiction (body) or obsession (mind), infatuation (other people), or mass hysteria (environments). At other times the surrender is voluntary, perhaps to something higher than the self. For someone with spiritual "ears to hear," this is God. For others, it is nature or art, their family or nation, their embattled sex or race, their ideology or profession.

Paradoxically, the human self may feel most truly itself when it has transcended the confines of the narrower self. As appears in the New Testament, it is by "losing" one's life that one "gains" it. The same may also apply to one's health.

*Hans Zinsser, *As I Remember Him: The Biography of R. S.*, Magnolia, Mass., Peter Smith Publisher, Inc., 1970.

For example, the characteristic IC pattern of Nobel scientist Andrei Sakarov and his wife, Elena Bonner, was to care more about human rights than about their own well-being. Yet despite their serious heart ailments, exacerbated by hunger strikes, they kept surviving to resist again another day. This pattern of strength—like its opposite—is usually visible to other people. "Isn't that just like Philip," a friend may say; or, to Philip himself, "How like you." Yet, on other occasions, Philip might comment, "I wasn't myself that day" (who, then, does he suppose he was?).

Another example of someone with a strong IC is writer Norman Cousins. Not only did he help himself recover from what was diagnosed as an incurable degenerative ailment of the connective tissue (ankylosing spondylitis), but seventeen years later, he also recovered from a severe heart attack. Though Cousins is unusual in his high degree of medical sophistication, his example can be useful to the average person (as is attested to by the popularity of his books, *Anatomy of an Illness: As Perceived by the Patient* and *The Healing Heart: Antidotes to Panic and Helplessness*). For one thing, he never gave up hope; for another, he never gave up the IC capacity to look at himself from a relatively objective point of view.

With the aid of his wife and doctors (other people), Cousins took control of his life and instituted changes (in his environments). Following the heart attack, he had a desk moved into his hospital room so that he could continue with his profession, writing. He asked for books and tapes that would make him laugh (mind and body), even though he had been warned that the physical effort of laughing might injure his weakened heart.

After his dismal results on the treadmill test, he refused to submit to another such test until he felt well enough to take control of the stop-start button. In time, his test results showed great improvement. How much was the result of his altered diet (no red meat, eggs, or cheese), his modified schedule (more time for rest and exercise), or the changes he had instituted in the testing procedure itself, no one knows. In any event, he recovered his good health sufficiently to go back to teaching doctors how, in effect, to take into account all four of a patient's health dimensions (as well as the intimate connector), rather than focusing solely on the dimension where the symptom first appears.

How many doctors, for example, think to ask a patient with abdominal pain, "How are you getting along with your relatives?" or "Is there something about your work place that's bothering you?"

Although American doctors, 70 percent of whom are specialists, may not show interest in all four of the patient's dimensions, the patient can learn to do so. No matter what the symptom, I can ask myself or someone

close to me, "What has changed—or is stubbornly resisting my worth-while attempts at change—in my:
• Body
• Mind
• Relationships with people
• Relationship with environments

As a patient reviews the state of each dimension, some clue may emerge that is worth bringing to the doctor's attention. The mother who bewails the flood that recently wrecked her ground floor may be helping the pediatrician get a fix on her child's unprecedented allergy. Even a clue that seems outlandish to the patient, such as the time of day or month or year when a symptom arose, is worth reporting. For, like Sherlock Holmes, the doctor is trained to look for seemingly irrelevant details that point toward accurate diagnosis. Patients, therefore, are better off pre-paring a too-long list of factual self-observations than a too-short one.

A man came to his internist with acute lower-back pain. The doctor prescribed bed rest and a muscle-relaxing drug.

"I guess I can't go to work?" the man remarked.

Something about the way he spoke made the doctor ask, "Is there any special tension in your shop?"

"Not at all. Last year there was, when the new guy was hired, but he's fitting in well enough."

"What's he doing?"

"I'm not exactly sure."

"Could he be angling for your job?"

"God! Wouldn't that be something! You know, the thought had crossed my mind."

"On your way home, why not stop by and ask the boss for a few minutes of his time. Everyone's turf needs redefining now and then. Maybe he can tell you what you'd like to hear."

"You mean that's why I'm all clenched up?"

"Could be. Besides, a fact of life is sometimes less hard on us than a fear we don't let ourselves face."

The man talked to his boss, was reassured, went home and climbed into bed. The pain, which might have taken two weeks to subside, dis-appeared in only two days.

Each health dimension comprises a vast number of parts and subparts that continually interact with each other and also with the parts and subparts of the other dimensions. One way to get a small handle on this never-ending process is through modern "systems thinking," a process based on the not-so-new observation that the whole can be greater than the sum of its parts.

What is new, though, is scientifically applying this whole-to-part relation to the management of health. As systems thinking demonstrates, if you change one part of a whole—or even *the relationship of one part to another*—you may change the whole. The patient who clarified his situation with his boss (other people) at the shop (environments) felt blessed relief (mind), which indirectly helped to lessen the spasm in his muscles (body).

Sometimes a person's four dimensions operate in a synergistic (mutually reinforcing) way, both for good and ill. Other times they serve to cancel each other out. But in general, when synergy occurs, a self-perpetuating health system—for good or ill—may get its start. This cycle, in turn, can develop an imposing momentum.

Good health, in short, is a wholesome cycle. I wake up feeling fine. I work or play; I relax alone or with a loved one in the evening; I sleep well and wake up feeling fine, perhaps even better.

Poor health is likely to be one of two things: either the merely temporary interruption of a characteristically wholesome cycle or the beginning of a vicious cycle. Because human health operates as an integrated system, a vicious cycle can be interrupted either in the dimension where the symptom first arose or *in any of the others*. The five main case histories in this book exemplify ways in which treatment in some dimension other than the original one may speed recovery.

Medicine is both a science and an art. The doctor who intuitively zeroed in on the patient's anxiety about his job was practicing medicine primarily as an art. The pathologist who studies slides, never so much as setting eyes on the patient whose name is on them, is practicing medicine primarily as a science.

A century and a half ago, medicine-as-science received a major impetus when improvements in the microscope opened up a new world of microbes and other forms of creation inconceivable through common sense alone. Excited by its new *un*common sense, medicine deliberately modeled itself on the work of physicists like Newton. The hypothesis was that for each event there must be an identifiable cause—one, it was hoped, that would also be measurable. When a specific germ was found in large number only in those patients with a particular disease, hope soared that what had worked so well for the physicists would work equally well for the physicians.

Indeed, everyone alive has reason to be grateful to the germ theory of disease and the immunizations and medications based upon it. Smallpox and polio, formerly capable of ruining or ending people's lives, have virtually been removed from the planet. Thanks to pioneering work by Jenner, Pasteur, Lister, Koch, Virchow, Enders, Sabin, and Salk, millions of people are now preventively spared infection by way of "the sanitary revolution" (i.e., potable water and milk, improved diet, efficient garbage disposal), vaccines, and medications.

At the same time, however, the one-eyed, or Cyclops, view of health— that there must be a single cause for each disease—was beginning to sow confusion. There were times when the *discoverable* cause of an ailment was not a *sufficient* cause. There were times when what *prolonged* the ailment was not what had *precipitated* it. With humans, more even than with microbes, much goes on that does not meet the eye—even the eye aided by the newest contact X-ray microscope.

In the realm of mind, as well as body, the discoverable cause was also turning out to be not necessarily the sufficient cause. Much, too, goes on that does not meet the psychiatrist's ear. Freud, for example, had assumed that one particular kind of unresolved childhood conflict was the cause of later paralysis (hysteria) in many of his patients. Yet some individuals were growing up symptom-free despite having suffered that specific early-life distress, while other people, after seemingly idyllic childhoods, were succumbing to hysterical paralysis and similar ills.

Around the turn of the century, some patients with *physical* symptoms, such as paralysis, were being diagnosed as having a *mental* illness. At the same time, some patients with *mental* symptoms, such as the delusions typical of paresis, were being diagnosed as having a *physical* illness (syphilis). To study this convertibility in both directions, a new branch of medicine arose in the 1920s. Named *psychosomatic medicine*, it postulated a direct, predictable bridge between soma (body) and psyche (mind and soul).

Early researchers were frustrated, however, when the emotional stress that triggered ulcers in Patient X, or hives in Patient Y, had no such effect on Person Z. In fact, so many simple psyche-to-soma experiments failed to show expected results that, by the 1950s, the new branch of medicine began losing professional adherents.

Ironically, around this time the public began embracing the psychosomatic concept. As a result, many patients felt guilty for their symptoms. "What am I doing wrong?" is still a question frequently asked of physicians. The frustrated doctors who, in more than half the cases cannot locate a clear, single, organic cause, may then guard their reputation for knowledgeability by allowing a patient to retain the impression that, yes, in some manner, he was at fault.

Patient guilt and anxiety were further heightened by computer printouts that linked some diseases with formerly innocuous habits, such as frequently eating bacon or serving it (many a middle-aged parent now feels like Lucretia Borgia). Yet much patient guilt remains misplaced and, if extreme, may itself become a health hazard. What such a patient needs is to view any risk he may have taken within the context of the huge multitude of influences on human health. Some of these are traceable, but many are not. So vast is their number and diversity of interaction with each other that even the most inclusive printout cannot begin to encompass them. Responsible scientists, therefore, have become far more tentative in their language. Instead of declaring A to be the *cause* of B, they call it a "risk factor" that "accompanies" B, or is "associated with" it. Indeed, some doctors, newly conscious of the complexities of illness, impatiently express disapproval of their patients' guilt, thus making them feel guilty for having felt guilty.

Much of the media continues to cast the blame for illness directly on patients. Even those citizens who have been trying valiantly to follow all the latest health rules (some of which contradict each other) are not exempt. Even that former symbol of wholesomeness, Mom's apple pie, has come under suspicion, as:

• environmentalists warn of the chemicals with which the apples may have been sprayed.
• cardiologists warn of the pie's salt, which may raise blood pressure, and butter and egg, which may increase cholesterol.
• dentists warn of the pie's sugar, which may erode teeth.
• and psychoanalysts warn of Mom.

More medical discoveries have been made in the past fifty years than in all of previous history. Small wonder that the professionals have trouble sorting them out, and that laypeople are bewildered. Whenever some new all-or-nothing health pronouncement is trumpeted, people do well to check it out with their own common sense and the experience of others. The language, too, offers helpful guidance in this regard, especially phrases like "on the one hand . . . and on the other" and "it all depends."

On the one hand, if I am exposed to virus X, I may catch the disease. *On the other hand*, if my exposure to it is neither frequent nor intense and if my immune defense system is working well, I may *not* catch the disease. *It all depends* on what else is going on at the time of the health event and what the components of that event may be.

Smokers who drink, for example, like drinkers who smoke, are far more likely to get cancer than people who have neither habit, or only one. (The chemical cause is probably ethyl nitrite, the production of which soars when alcohol and smoke are held in the mouth at the same time.)*

Still, not every smoker, even those who drink, gets cancer. *It all depends* on the individual's heredity and temperament, IC strength, home life, habits of work and play, and whether the multitude of factors in his various dimensions happen to dovetail most of the time into a wholesome or vicious cycle.

Although the step that halts or reverses a vicious cycle is often a minor one, *not* to take this—or some other—helpful step may permit the cycle's natural momentum to mount. Take, for example, the worker with the bad back. Had he *not* been started on a wholesome cycle by his doctor's advice, instead forcing himself to keep going despite the increasing severity of his pain, he might well have come home in such a state that he proceeded to:
• drink too much (body).
• sink into gloom (mind).
• turn against his spouse or children (relationships with people).
• storm out of the house despite a storm (relationship with environments).
• feel miserably at war with himself (IC).

Any one of these steps might have made his back worse, perhaps in turn causing him to engage in another of the steps, until he ended up totally incapacitated.

A clear description of health momentum in both the wholesome and vicious directions appears in the New Testament: "Unto everyone that hath shall be given . . . but from him that hath not, shall be taken away even that which he hath."

Unfair? Indeed, yes. But so is the distribution of good health, both as between one person and another, and also, within the same person, as between one stage of life and another.

For the lucky individual with good genes and a well-functioning IC, to remain fit takes little effort: It is "doin' a-what comes naturally."† For someone less fortunate, or at a less "together" stage, a minor ailment in one dimension may set in motion troublesome reactions in other di-

*Smoke-a-holics may be jarred by Peter Taylor's comment in *The Smoke Ring* that, in effect, smoking "has wiped out more people than all the wars of this century." And even mild smokers may be jarred by the 1985 results of the thirty-year cardiovascular study in Framingham, Massachusetts, funded by The National Institutes of Health. According to its director, William P. Castelli, M.D., "For every cigarette smoked each day, the risk of lung cancer increases one time over the risk faced by nonsmokers. Thus, someone who smoked five cigarettes a day is five times more likely to get lung cancer than a nonsmoker." (*New York Times*, 8 January 1985).
†"Fit," according to one of its Middle English roots, means "together." Current phrases, such as "getting my act (or head) together," are, therefore, right on target.

mensions. Some vicious cycles, moreover, may continue not only for the rest of that person's life but on down through the generations. As was noted in the Old Testament, "The fathers have eaten a sour grape and the children's teeth are set on edge." A heart-rending example is the battered child who grows up to batter his own children.

Sometimes a vicious cycle needs to be interrupted by oneself or a relative, a friend or doctor, not only because the symptoms are painful but also because the cycle's momentum has become like a broken window in an abandoned house: a stimulus to further destruction.

Why? Why do some people "become their own worst enemy"? Why would any reasonable individual, as Oscar Wilde poignantly generalized from his own downward spiral, "kill the thing he loves?"

Yet some highly intelligent people, not excluding doctors, develop so much momentum in an *intra*personal cycle that it engages their *inter*personal ones. One of the latter may then ricochet back into the intra-personal realm, with the baffling result that is referred to as "a self-fulfilling prophecy" or "creating the very thing he fears."

For example, a wife, troubled by migraine and deep insecurities, worried that her husband would wander. She watched him so closely that after a while he began to fear for his independence and manhood. Eventually he took up with a more symptom-free and trusting partner. This, in turn, increased the wife's migraines and insecurities. . . .

On the one hand, no one knows the near-infinite number of times when an ailment has been forestalled—or prevented from becoming serious—by someone's having eased up on his own schedule, or his demands on someone else. Certainly no one need worry about an occasional "bad day" when he feels below par or keeps saying or doing the wrong thing. Perhaps he is expressing some buried anger that he has not yet come to grips with, or perhaps the sunspots and electromagnetic waves from outer space are roiling his internal rhythms. In any event, it is only when a self-destructive *pattern* appears in his health that his IC, perhaps with the help of a doctor, needs to institute a change in one or more of his dimensions. If a particular change does not work, there are a multitude of others to be tried, as, over what is hoped will be a long and active lifetime, he proceeds to *get* well, *stay* well, and—though different from the other two, equally important—*feel* well.

DR. TAMARKIN: I hope our readers will sympathize with some of the five patients we've chosen to illustrate the four dimensions and the IC.

JUNE BINGHAM: I could cheerfully throttle those patients.

NORMAN: That doesn't seem very charitable.

JUNE: It's *not*. But they're driving me crazy in terms of the book's organization. Like Procrustes' guests, they will *not* fit into the bed prepared for them. Take Sanford, whose physical symptoms make him suitable for our chapter on *body*. But what does he end up needing? Help with his *psyche*?

NORMAN: Sanford is typical of almost a third of the patients who seek general health care. What really helps them is some form of psychiatric intervention. Thank goodness, physicians—and some patients, too—have begun to realize this.

JUNE: Or Mary Ellen, the semisuicidal young woman who's suitable for our chapter on *mind*: what does she do but improve because of antibiotics, better nutrition, and exercise?

NORMAN: That, too, is typical of lots of patients. Until their body can be brought into better condition, they can't summon enough energy for the hard work of uncovering the emotional conflicts that underlie their symptoms to begin with.

JUNE: Readers need to know that's why the cases don't just stop at the end of their respective chapters, but are continued throughout the book.

NORMAN: Also, that while the *facts* about each of these people are accurate, their *interrelationships* are invented. In real life, each person had someone close to him who is *like* the fellow patient in the book but *is* not, in fact, that person.

JUNE: Maybe we'd better admit that although one case is a success, one is sort of a failure, and the other three fall somewhere in between.

NORMAN: All of which reflects the state of the art.

JUNE: How well does holistic medicine fit into your "art"?

NORMAN: Many aspects of holism are valuable, but so are many aspects of traditional medicine. At times, the one can be used as a valuable corrective for the other.

JUNE: Where do you, personally, agree and disagree with them?

NORMAN: You don't mind asking broad questions, do you?

JUNE: Why should I? It's not every day that a layperson gets a psychiatrist in the position where he has to answer one's questions.

NORMAN: Okay. Holistic medicine is a type of practice where the professional persuades his patients to modify their social and ecological environments, as well as their physical and mental states. Holistic practitioners also help the patient and his family understand the day-to-day progress of the illness. Medical information is not kept secret from them. While I agree that much of modern medicine needs to be "demystified," I disagree when holistic practitioners rely on unproved dietary supplements or megadoses of approved ones. Not only might these do the patient harm, but they may prevent him from taking the traditional measures that would do him good. I also disagree with proponents of holism who blame what they call our "sick society" for everything bad that happens to the individual. Dr. Thomas Szasz, a medical iconoclast, for example, relies so thoroughly on *social* causation that he denies the existence of any *individual* mental illness.

JUNE: What about the holistic people who have a healthier-than-thou attitude?

NORMAN: A great mistake. Health is not a competitive sport. I also part company with them when they say that if you just "live right"—and the definition of *that* changes every few years—you'll "defeat" illness and maintain "wellness" until you die at a very old age. That's just not the way health works out when the individual is living a long full life.

JUNE: What do you think of traditional medicine?

NORMAN: Well, obviously, the scientific method has given us some extraordinary health miracles. You, with your repaired spine, and I, with my repaired heart, are walking examples. But some doctors hold their medical knowledge too close to their chest. And some hospitals buy wildly expensive modern equipment they don't really need. And to make it pay for itself, their doctors may overuse it. Another weakness of traditional medicine is in the field of diet. When I was at medical school, there was only one half-year course on the subject. Lots of traditional doctors know less about nutrition than some of their patients do. And they know even less about holistic practices of possible effectiveness, such as acupuncture.

JUNE: Will the two types of medicine ever get together?

NORMAN: There are areas where they must! A responsible holistic doctor who suspects a patient has cancer shouldn't hesitate to refer him to a traditional practitioner of oncology or radiology for diagnosis or treatment. Similarly, a responsible radiologist, faced with too many patients to get to know them very well, shouldn't hesitate to refer a cancer patient who's been through the traditional treatments to a reputable holistic center for advice about food, exercise, massage, or meditation. But whether a patient relies on holistic or traditional advice, or some combination of the two, he should ultimately be the captain of his own health ship. Sure, he needs to take aboard a doctor as pilot when the waves of poor health build up, but it is the patient who should take the responsibility for his own well-being, the quality of his living, and the form of his dying.

JUNE: I bet a lot of doctors would take issue with you.

NORMAN: They do.

II
New Perspectives on Health

Introducing Martha

*"The desire to take medicine is perhaps the greatest
feature which distinguishes man from animals."*
—Sir William Osler

Martha, an elderly underweight woman, was brought to the hospital's emergency room by the superintendent of her building. She had a high fever and was semidelirious.

The diagnosis was bronchial pneumonia. Before antibiotics, this disease carried off so many of its suffering elderly hosts that it was nicknamed "the old man's friend." But today, with treatment, most people recover.

Martha was placed in a small ward without windows. She refused all food and, despite intravenous antibiotics every four hours, her temperature remained high. When her daughter, Dorothy, appeared, Martha greeted her by name but said nothing further. Distraught, Dorothy went to fetch her father, Peter, who had been on bad terms with Martha since their divorce long ago. When he sat down at the bedside, laid a hand on her arm, and tried to tell her he was sorry, Martha grimaced and turned her face to the wall. Peter stamped out. Dorothy stayed for several more hours. At ten o'clock, exhausted, she went home. Late in the night, Martha died.

The cause of death was listed as pneumonia. Dorothy, herself a nurse, insisted on an autopsy. The pneumonia must have been viral, not bacterial, she argued; why else would the antibiotic have had no effect? But the pneumonia was not viral. What neither Dorothy nor the busy doctors had taken into account was the likelihood that Martha might have been suffering from depression (mind) or that, because of her long-term loneliness (relationships with other people), she had lost her will to live (IC).

Her thinness might have reflected a long-term disinterest in food (body), and her hospital room's lack of window (environment) might have contributed to her inability to heal (statistics now point to daylight as one of many variables that speed recovery).

Thus, as often happens, the assumption of a single, quantifiable, laboratory-verifiable cause served to obscure other, perhaps equally, or even more, significant causes.

Nan Robertson, a well-known journalist, had the opposite type of experience, and survived to write about it in a Pulitzer prize–winning article.* She was fifty-five when toxic shock attacked all her vital organs. Every resource of the hospital's intensive care unit was needed to keep her feeble flicker of life from going out. Later, because of uncontrollable gangrene, eight of her fingers had to be partially amputated. "If anybody had a good reason to die," her doctor told her, "you did. Your age alone! If you had been a fifteen- or twenty-year-old, it wouldn't be so unusual. Of course this just means you're tough as nails."

A nurse at the Howard A. Rusk Institute for Rehabilitation at New York University Medical Center phrased it differently: "There are the survivors, and there are those who would rather . . . just slip under. All human beings divide into these two groups. I have even seen babies who do not want to live—who literally pined away and died."

In addition to her strong IC and the prompt, expert medical care she was given, Nan Robertson had support from devoted family, friends, and working colleagues. Nonetheless, she, like Martha, was suffused with inchoate rage: "As soon as they took me off the respirator, I began to heap my anger onto my family, the doctors, and nurses. I reviled everyone who entered the room. . . . For at least ten days I was possessed by fury, at everyone. One morning I awoke . . . cleansed and filled with hope. 'You have everything to live for,' I told myself. That morning . . . my recovery truly began. It has been a long road back."

Although the difficult years that followed caused her to rage at her own helplessness and the constant presence of pain, she was willing to make the requisite effort for rehabilitation. As she finally concluded, "There is no way to win at physical therapy without working through pain to healing."

Healing is what the patient tries to do; curing is what the doctor tries to do. When these two efforts mesh, the result can be magnificent. Yet

*Nan Robertson, "Toxic Shock," *The New York Times Magazine,* 19 September 1982.

until the 1930s, when sulfa drugs first came into use, doctors were not able to do much to cure most illnesses except pay frequent and palliative house calls. For in their little black bags they carried nothing that could counter the tuberculosis, rheumatic fever, smallpox, diphtheria, or tetanus, which were the chief killers in the United States until the turn of the century. With the serious *mental* ills, doctors could do even less. Patients, in effect, had to get well on their own.

The most dramatic contemporary breakthrough in doctor-instigated cure came in the 1940s with the discovery of antibiotics. Rapid recovery from numerous ills could be accomplished by even the least experienced physician. Sometimes he did not even need to see the patient but prescribed over the phone a pill that could reduce the patient's fever (from, say, bronchial pneumonia) from 104 to 98 degrees within hours.

In the 1950s, the serious mental ills, too, came within the doctors' curative scope. New mood-altering (psychotropic) and other drugs brought marvelous relief. A schizophrenic patient who for years had been on a back ward, neither speaking nor appearing to know where he was, was given chlorpromazine. One day he approached the doctor. "Excuse me, sir, but could you tell me why you are keeping me in this dismal place? I feel perfectly all right." And he *was* relatively all right, although, like Rip Van Winkle, he had problems adjusting to a world that had gone on without him. Fortunately, his IC was strong enough to keep him taking his medication after he left the hospital.

Yet another development came in the early 1970s, when computer analysis began revealing how influential some of a person's habits and attitudes are on his health. Thus did the pendulum of health responsibility swing back to the patient, not only for getting well but also for not getting sick to begin with.

In one sense, therefore, there were only about four decades, roughly from 1930 to 1970, when, overall, doctors were perceived as doing more for their patients' health than the patients, with a combination of good medical advice and common sense, could do for themselves.

Furthermore, drawbacks to prevailing professional practice began being publicized. One new issue was the dangerous side effects of some drugs, either solo or in combination. The term *iatrogenic* was coined to refer to ailments caused by doctors (thalidomide babies being a tragic example). With an average of three new drugs coming on the market daily (one thousand per year), even specialists have trouble keeping up with all their ramifications. Particularly with the psychotropic drugs, is it important that the doctor dispensing them be up to date on their direct effects, side effects, and interactions with other drugs and nutrients.

Medical specialties themselves are also on the increase. If today we have otology (the study of ears) and oncology (the study of cancer), pediatrics (the study of children) and podiatry (the study of feet), tomorrow we will probably have the specialty of pediatric otological (or podriatal) oncology.

Another new kind of health problem relates to the harmful effects of some otherwise useful technologies, such as radiology. The term *nosocomial* was coined to describe ailments caused by inappropriate use of such technologies or other forms of negligence by hospitals.

Still another type of problem occurs when a patient runs up against conflicting advice from specialists. Though each physician is conscientiously tending to the aspect of the patient's health he knows most about, the two doctors often neglect to coordinate their advice. One brand-new mother, for example, was ordered by her orthopedist to start up her back exercises right away, and by her obstetrician to avoid exertion for the first few weeks. In the end, it was she who decided which doctor to obey. Later she was told she should have phoned her internist to ask him to adjudicate between the other two. Sometimes, in fact, the patient's decision about whether or not to consult a doctor, and if so, what kind, may be the most important component in recovery of good health.

The feeling of well-being is connected not only to one's actual state of health but also to one's ability to manufacture, in various parts of brain or body, minute quantities of homegrown painkillers and mood-lifters. Endorphins (meaning literally "like morphine") are one such group of neurochemicals. No one knows how to produce more of them *directly*: were they to be eaten or injected, the body would simply digest them. But *indirectly*, by way of the four dimensions and the IC, their supply may be deliberately increased:

- By the *body*, via exercise. Research shows that higher levels of endorphins are produced and maintained by regular exercisers than by sedentary types.
- By the *mind*, via meditation; or appreciation of music, art, literature, theater, film, television, or games.
- By relationships with *people*, through words of appreciation or a gentle touch, given or received.
- By relationship with one's *environments*, through immersing oneself in nature or community activity.
- By the *IC*, through the sense of mastery that derives from choosing a desirable goal that one is capable of achieving, and then achieving it.

Recent experiments at the National Institutes of Health by Drs. Michael R. Ruff and Candace Pert indicate that there is a link between one of the endorphins and a major cell of the immune system (the macrophage). Earlier research had pointed to a link between aspects of brain chemistry and the hormone-producing glands that also can affect the immune system. What this suggests is that a circular series of reactions takes place that can guard or restore good health, with the brain directly or indirectly affecting the immune and hormone systems, which themselves affect the brain.

The relationship between endorphins and the IC also appears to be circular. This may help to explain the mutual reinforcement that sometimes occurs between happiness and good health. Take the contrast between one couple who effortlessly bask in each other's company and hardly ever have a sick day, and another couple, of similar age and circumstance, who strain to keep one roof over their two heads while suffering hives or headaches, depression or digestive upset. No sooner, moreover, is one of their ailments alleviated than another one erupts.

An IC-endorphin cycle may be involved in a further paradox—namely, the ability some people have to devote themselves to a purpose more significant than themselves, even to the point of abusing their health, yet end up in better shape than other people who think of little *except* their health. At the same time, some people devoted to jogging and dieting may unconsciously be reflecting an IC urge, during our chaotic era, to establish control over at least one area of personal accomplishment, and thus indirectly add to their IC strength and supply of endorphins.

Among the most puzzling relationships is the paradoxical one between health and virtue. While some people sicken because of doing the medically *forbidden* thing, such as eating too many animal fats, others sicken because of doing the morally or medically *recommended* thing, such as dedicating themselves to the care of a dying relative or friend. Even in ancient Greece, the dramatist Menander observed that "whom the gods love dies young," while in ancient Israel the psalmist deplored the other side of the same coin, namely, "the wicked flourishing like a green bay tree."

Today, the possible health hazards that accompany some types of extreme virtue are being taken into account. For example, an overly acquiescent child or a compulsive overachiever may cause more concern to doctor, teacher, or parent than does the average young rascal, who gets a lift out of his own mischief.*

In fact, some old adages and moral edicts are being reevaluated from the point of view of their health impact. Leo Rotan, a psychiatric social worker, found in a survey that a large number of male heart-attack victims,

---

*One theory about the cause of anorexia nervosa is that the self-starvers, 90 percent of whom are female, are symbolically striving for perfection. Another theory is that the anorexic patient is unconsciously acting out her *family's* unrealistic fantasies about perpetual improvement.

aged thirty to seventy, believed that "a winner never quits; a quitter never wins," while, in a matched group free from heart attack, a large number believed that "life is just a bowl of cherries."*

A major moral edict that has withstood the tests of time and modern medicine is the commandment to love one's neighbor *and* oneself. One that has failed the tests is the prohibition against saying bad things about people behind their backs. Indeed, much of psychotherapy could be defined as precisely such articulation of disloyalty. Patients are encouraged to report to their doctor or therapy group about key people in their lives. At the same time, they are encouraged to explore and perhaps relive, within this artificially safe environment, the most wounding moments in their previous relationships. After having done so, they often find a way to reverse an old vicious cycle they might not previously have been aware of as such. Perhaps, for instance, my defensive attitude toward someone has caused me to act in a stiff manner that, in turn, elicited the kind of displeasure from him that caused my defensive behavior in the first place.

Even without a doctor or therapy group, people can use what has been called "controlled disloyalty" as an aid to better health. If there is someone in my life who is "making me sick" or "driving me crazy" and I can complain to you about him, I may, first of all, feel the better for having ventilated my resentment. Second, I may feel the better for your acceptance of my complaint as neither sick, crazy, nor wicked. Third, I may profit from your rational response, which broadens my IC's angle of vision, thus enabling me to view the offender and myself as parts of a larger whole.

Some marriage counselors, for example, ask the partners to consider, in addition to their individual needs, those of the marriage itself. Is *it* being strengthened or weakened by, say, their customary environment for substantive discussion? If talking in the bedroom keeps broadening the fissures in the relationship, perhaps the kitchen would be better. Or if the kitchen is viewed as too much one partner's turf, then maybe the living room or the outdoors is a better place. By and large, the more neutral the surroundings, the easier the two-way communication. On the other hand, as also in parent-child and intersibling relationships, a cordial visit by the more secure partner to the turf of the less secure one may itself add to the health of the relationship. This, in turn, may expand the IC perspectives of both the individuals concerned.

The idea of cajoling—or jolting—an individual into feeling better by

*A staff-written article, "Can Proverbs Cause Heart Attacks?" in *Science Digest*, April, 1982.

suggesting a change in some dimension other than the one where the symptom first made its appearance is not intrinsically new. In the last century it was routine for doctors or friends to advise patients to "take the waters" or "get a change of air" or, for women, to "go out and buy a new hat." But the advice was generally not incorporated into any overall health philosophy.

Today, a health philosophy, like contemporary physics and mathematics, is less likely to be based on certainties than on statistical probabilities. It also needs to make room for exceptions to these probabilities. And exceptions occur far more frequently with humans than with electrons or quanta. Why? Because, in addition to the human complexity, uniqueness, and freedom, there is also the factor referred to as fate, or God's will, or happenstance, or just plain luck. Napoleon, when presented with the name of a general for a crucial campaign, would ask, "A-t'il de la chance?" ("Is he lucky?").

In estimating whether some health probability will apply to ourselves, we need to consider, in addition to "luck," our vital statistics at that time. Not only do individuals differ from one another in their response to foods and drugs, but they also differ from *themselves* at an earlier or later age. What "agrees with" someone when young may disagree with him when he is old, or vice versa.

A less obvious factor is the individual's mood and IC power on a given day. Sometimes we enjoy taking a risk, and we get away with it, even feel the better for it. Other times we had best lie low: too many occasions for self-blame that day. In addition to people's apparent accident-proneness, freak accidents can happen: a brick may fall off a roof onto someone's head. Other times, what appears to be an accident is a part of some unconscious pattern of one's own.

Semantic confusion surrounding the word *accident* compounds the problem. It is used to refer to an injury that is *self*-caused ("I accidentally fell off my bike") and also for an injury caused by *others* ("it was an accident; she didn't mean to spill coffee on me"). The word is even used in the sense of "accidentally-on-purpose" (a concept colorfully elaborated on by Freud in *The Psychopathology of Everyday Life*). An example would be a child who is forced by his parents to become a violinist but who "accidentally" mashes his fingers in a door. The term *accident-prone*, therefore, should ideally be altered to *injury-prone*, since some investigation may be necessary before discovering whether there was an *outer* cause for a *true* accident or an *inner* cause for what is then really *not* accidental at all.

In either event, an IC overview by oneself or another person may be useful. A child who keeps falling and hurting himself may have a middle-ear infection that impairs his balance (body). Or he may always feel in a hurry (mind). Or he may be craving affection from parents who rarely make time for him except when he is incapacitated (relationships with other people). Or the floors of his home may simply have been too well polished (relationship with environments). After objectively weighing the factors, a change in one dimension or another may bring about an improved result.

For example, a woman was taken aback when her husband asked, "Do you realize that it's always a week before your period when you trip over things and scold the kids for being so sloppy?" When she consulted her calendar, she found he was right. She reported this to her doctor. After trying several medications, he gave her a diuretic. This drained excess fluid from her tissues, including those of the brain. No longer badgered by an extreme irritability that she had been blaming on her children but that was really part of premenstrual syndrome (PMS),* she felt better and was more patient with her family, who, in turn, responded by behaving more as she had hoped.

Because of these elements—chance, the freedom and uniqueness of the individual, and the degree of IC involvement at a particular time—people often end up surprising their doctor. Sometimes a genetically transmitted ailment turns up in one identical twin but not in the other; sometimes it turns up in both but cripples only one. In short, to "luck out" in terms of health, one need not have had flawless parents, nor live in a garden spot in uninterrupted harmony with angelic companions, nor follow the latest health fad.

To get sick, furthermore, may—or may not—offer the opportunity to learn something useful for next time (specific forms of health advice are included in Appendices A through G). Sometimes the patient had been too cavalier, overworking or overplaying and not heeding the early warning signals from body or mind or relationships. But at other times, the patient's behavior had been exemplary. Even so, he may not be able to relax and enjoy his episode of minor ill health because he is so unstrung by all the warnings in the media about self-inflicted doom. For example, three of the *better* than ordinary books in recent years were entitled *The Save-Your-Life Diet* (eat bran, or else!); *Kill Stress Before It Kills You* (meditate, or else!); and *Mind the Healer, Mind the Slayer* (learn biofeedback, or else!). Put together with the many less responsible outpourings, the cumulative result has been that Americans, a people formerly

*Whether the law should take PMS into account in sentencing women for violent crimes is passionately debated. In England, the law does permit the PMS argument, but in the United States, feminist groups, among others, oppose it. As to PMS causes and the effectiveness of various treatments, there remains a great deal of controversy.

known for their optimism, are currently described as "the worried well" and "the healthy hypochondriacs." Fortunately, some typically American spoofs have also appeared, such as the bumper-sticker announcing that "*Living* Causes Cancer" and Richard Smith's book *The Dieter's Guide to Weight Loss During Sex.*

A nonjudgmental doctor may, therefore, be offering to his sick patient a form of relief more soothing than the heat-pad or ice-pack or prescribed medication. Indeed, the very concept of "no-fault illness" can be a spur to better health, whether communicated by the doctor or someone else who says, "Oh well, these things happen." In the United States, recognition of no-fault illness may also serve to mitigate the British tradition of "stiff upper lip" that encourages some people to delay for too long their admission that something is wrong with them. Somehow, to be caught suffering seems un-American; as the British historian Arnold Toynbee once observed, "In the U.S. it is unfashionable to die."

Yet animals in the wild often suffer from cancer and heart disease, true accidents and fits of irrational behavior. An occasional period of ill health is a fact of nature. The chief advantage for humans is that, when ailing, we are less likely to be eaten by a predator; the chief advantage for animals is that they are less likely to be eaten by guilt.

JUNE: So you don't advise anyone to try to achieve perfect health?

NORMAN: No. In fact, I think it's a mistake to take any diet or exercise program too far.

JUNE: Why?

NORMAN: Obsessive dieting can spoil the person's digestion and also other people's enjoyment at table. Obsessive running can injure a man's joints—maybe even his marriage.

JUNE: How?

NORMAN: He's on the road too much.

JUNE: Can a *doctor* be too conscientious about a patient's health?

NORMAN: Sometimes. If your doctor orders an invasive test, like putting a catheter into a vein, on the off chance of finding some unlikely evidence of disease, you should say, "Hey, wait a minute. Isn't being ninety-eight percent certain good enough? Why, at the risk of injuring me, try for a hundred percent?"

JUNE: Yet the doctor will probably preface his ordering of the test by saying, "Let's do this just to be on the *safe* side," while real safety might mean to avoid the test—or the doctor.

NORMAN: Some doctors are so scared of malpractice suits that they routinely order every test in the book for every patient. Yet some of these tests are both painful and possibly dangerous, and surely expensive.

JUNE: So there are trade-offs in medicine that the patient should be aware of.

NORMAN: Not only about tests, but drugs and operations. Take, for example, the postmenopausal woman who is advised to take estrogen. If she is lucky, this female hormone may help her avoid osteoporosis, the brittleness of bone that has become almost epidemic in older American women; if she is unlucky, she may develop a cancer of the uterus.

JUNE: But that means she'd need a hysterectomy. Aren't far too many of those being performed?

NORMAN: Yes. But still, she has a choice. Which is worse from the point of view of her future? An eventual broken hip that may *not* heal, or, long before that, an operation that *will* heal? Also, she and the doctor need to review whether her mother, grandmother, sister, and aunt have, or have not, been cancer-prone. And she must, even if she's on the lightest doses of estrogen, go for a checkup every six to twelve months. Endometrial cancer can be diagnosed very early.

JUNE: What if she and the doctor disagree?

NORMAN: She should ask for a second opinion. Even if she and the doctor do agree about an operation, she should ask for a second opinion. But in either event, it's important for her to feel free to express her feelings to her doctor. I'm a great believer in the inherent chemistry between doctor and patient. When a patient truly trusts her doctor and is open with him, she empowers the doctor to help her to an extraordinary degree. And then, of course, the doctor feels great too!

JUNE: You mean that *two* IC-endorphin cycles get swinging between doctor and patient?

NORMAN: In any kind of relationship. My patients and I frequently draw interlocking circles that identify a wholesome—or vicious—cycle in one dimension triggering minicycles in other dimensions, both within the patient and between him and other people.

JUNE: What's an example?

NORMAN: Take Martha, the pneumonia patient. Her daughter Dorothy was what we call the SO.

JUNE: What does that stand for?

NORMAN: The "significant other": the relative or friend who really matters to the patient. In fact, if the doctor and the SO can work well in harness, they may accomplish far more than either could on his own.

JUNE: What should the SO do?

NORMAN: Mostly just be there for the patient—sometimes to offer a smile or word of encouragement, sometimes a funny bit of news or a simple touch. Some patients, especially in intensive care units, are touched only by machines, not people. They may become what is now called "skin-starved."

JUNE: But Peter tried to touch Martha.

NORMAN: Hard to say about Martha's response to him. Some patients are invigorated by their hatred; others are weakened by it. There's nothing like a surge of righteous wrath—or even *un*-righteous wrath—to propel someone out of a sickbed.

JUNE: But Martha didn't rally.

NORMAN: Still, she wasn't indifferent. There was strong emotion that could have been worked with, if there had been a doctor who knew her well enough.

JUNE: Or a nurse?

NORMAN: Very much so. The nurse often gets to know the patient better than the doctor does.

JUNE: What about knowing the family members?

NORMAN: That can be very useful. To get a variety of perspectives on the patient is sometimes necessary because *being* sick and *feeling* sick aren't always the same thing. At one end of the continuum is the patient who is objectively dying of TB but subjectively confident he's getting better. At the other end is the person whose objective tests all show up normal yet subjectively continues to feel rotten.

JUNE: Is he likely to be in a depression?

NORMAN: Not really. A clinically depressed person feels that same lack of zest, but to a far more extreme degree. Also, his despair is accompanied by other symptoms.

JUNE: Such as?

NORMAN: Insomnia, indecision, weight loss, crippling anxiety (especially in the mornings), sometimes closeness to tears, sometimes fantasies, even talk, of suicide. But what doctors run into all the time is the patient who isn't really depressed but is operating like a car on only one cylinder.

JUNE: What should such people do?

NORMAN: Get their IC into the act and determine that they are going to regain and maintain and enjoy good health. They should carefully choose a doctor and bring him a "laundry list" of what's going on in all four of their dimensions. This is the realm of medicine where the patient can be of most help to the doctor. Also, sometimes, the doctor's reassurance that he feels enthusiastic about becoming a health partner to this patient is enough to reverse an old cycle of patient fear leading to inner clenching and thus to further fear. With this partial lifting of the patient's burden, the patient may be more resistant to future health hazards. The hormones, the immune system, and the endorphins are like the chicken and the egg. We can't yet prove which comes first, but if you get either one going in the right direction, you may start up a wholesome momentum in the other.

III
Mostly Body

Introducing Sanford

"A medical symptom may be a useful signal of the need for change in other parts of the person's life."
—Kenneth R. Pelletier

At thirty, Sanford was a big man, six feet five. He weighed 250 pounds, but much of it was muscle from the basketball he played several nights a week. His fiancée, Esmé, teasingly complained that he pursued the basketball more avidly than her.

On basketball evenings, he would eat lightly. But other times he and Esmé might have three belts of whiskey before dinner and a bottle of red wine with their rare roast beef. Esmé tried to get Sanford to eat the salad ("It's free, after all"). But he either ignored it or doused it with blue-cheese dressing ("That's free too").

He gave up cigars because Esmé did not like the smell, but he smoked two to three packs of cigarettes a day.

His job as a salesmen for a restaurant-equipment company involved a lot of driving. He liked to speed, weaving in and out of traffic. But one day, after a near miss, he began to feel dizzy. The dizziness went away, but the memory of it did not. He scheduled a physical exam.

The doctor was no-nonsense. "Lose fifty pounds and quit smoking."

"You have to be kidding. No one can do both at the same time."

"If you want to live to a ripe old age, you'll find a way."

"I don't care about living forever. I like living it up right now."

The doctor shrugged. "Don't say I didn't warn you."

"Or *hex* me!"

Though Sanford cut back on eating and smoking, his worry about himself increased. His sleep became fitful, and stabs of pain came and went in his left shoulder, back, and chest. He said nothing to

Esmé; what was not admitted might go away. But he drank more.

When Esmé pointed out that the calories in booze put as much weight on you as those in food, he told her to quit being such a spoilsport. Gradually he gained back the pounds he had lost; gradually the cigarette tally climbed up again.

One night, he felt his heart palpitate when he lay down—and he was frightened. "Beginning to feel my age," he told Esmé.

"Me, too," she said. "If I'm ever going to have kids, we'd better get married pretty soon."

Again his heart took a jolt—but he smiled and patted her.

A few days later, he was driving more aggressively than usual. The dizziness returned. This time it did not, as he expected, go away. He realized he had to slow down—in every sense. When the road's shoulder became wider, he pulled off. He could scarcely breathe, so much was his heart pounding and hurting. He laid his head down on the wheel.

A siren. For a moment, he thought he was still speeding and the cops were after him. Flashing red lights. "What's the trouble, mister?" Soon he was in an ambulance—and then in a hospital bed. He felt deep relief. He had done his best. Now all responsibility was out of his hands.

Tests and more tests. Esmé came. "You relax about the wedding," she said. "We'll see how you feel in six months."

Blessed relief. He did not want to make any decisions. But then fear. Perhaps *she* didn't want *him*. Why would anyone want to marry an invalid? Two years before, when he had proposed to her, she had said she wanted to think about it. Two months ago, when she had said she was ready, he'd been the one to postpone setting a date. He enjoyed his freedom to go out with the boys for drinks after basketball, and not having to earn a lot of money. But when Esmé began mentioning that she'd had lunch with a male colleague, Sanford felt a wild surge of jealousy. He couldn't bear the thought of her dating someone else, yet he was frightened at the prospect of supporting a family. He would need a raise. What if the boss turned him down? Should he quit his job? Maybe Esmé should quit *hers*, and get away from that son of a bitch who took her out to lunch. How dare he muscle in on Sanford's girl? Yet who could blame Esmé for wanting a child? He wouldn't love her so much if she didn't yearn to be a mother. Yet did *he* want to be a father? Might he, God forbid, end up like his own father, the admiral, barking orders at home as if on shipboard, paralyzing his kids with fear?

One morning the doctor came and sat by Sanford's bed. "You've got two problems. One is a mild form of diabetes. The other is a mild form of heart irregularity, what we call cardiac arrhythmia. Luckily, your heart hasn't suffered any damage—and your diabetes will be controllable by diet."

"Then why do you look so grim?"

"Because you're not going to like what I have to say."

"Go ahead. I can take it."

"I think you should see a psychiatrist."

"*What?*"

"You're under some kind of emotional stress. You and I are not equipped to spot what it is. But something is making your heart take extra beats; something is interfering with your pancreas, so it isn't turning out enough insulin."

"But—"

"I can help you manage your symptoms with medication, but you need a psychiatrist to help you find out why you developed them to begin with."

"How can a shrink do anything for my heart and pancreas?"

"By helping you uncover some underlying emotional conflict that you don't know much about."

"If *I* don't know about it, how the hell can *you?*"

"Because of your heart that misbehaves and your diabetes. Those are two symptoms that sometimes call for psychotherapy."

"I don't see why!"

"Look, Sanford. When people feel under threat, they release adrenaline into their bloodstream. Even the tiniest drop of it speeds the heart and slows the pancreas. Your glucose-tolerance tests show that your sugar goes up too fast and stays up too long. If the doctor can help you identify whatever you're responding to as if it were a current threat, then your symptoms will improve."

"If you and that damn shrink don't drive me crazy first."

Sanford broke his first three appointments with the psychiatrist. Finally he did go, and complained of heart pain, dizziness, and constant terror of dying. He was now so afraid of having a heart attack some place where help couldn't reach him that he had worked out elaborate new routes to his customers, routes lined with stores and gas stations. It took longer and used up more gas.

Later sessions with the doctor were sometimes cut short when Sanford clutched his chest and walked in gingerly fashion to the office of his internist in the same building, in order to have an electrocardiogram. But only small irregularities if any, every showed up.

As the psychiatrist said later, "Because Sanford is a rough-tough macho type, I recognized how hard it was for him to talk with another man about intimate details. Whenever the conversation approached the tangled mix of feelings he has about his family, he would shout, 'Bullshit!' He preferred to talk about his fears of losing his health, even his life. Because of his heart symptoms, he has totally given up cigarettes, and he is dieting. But he claims that the joy has gone out of everything. He is terrified of losing his job and, most of all, his fiancée. 'She has a strong nesting instinct,' he says. 'She can't wait forever for me to get well.' "

Sanford is the middle child, with an older brother and younger sister. During their childhood, the navy moved the family every few years. Sanford was big, fat, and clumsy, and the other boys picked on him. They would grab his books or throw away his pencils. On occasion, he was forced to fight. He reports that he never lost a fight except against his older brother, who outdid him in every way. Peaceable by nature, Sanford could battle hard when he had to. Indeed, he sometimes frightened himself with the violence of his feelings.

Sanford still visits his parents one Sunday a month, but he does not feel close to them. Though retired, his father continues to bark out orders, and Sanford's mother and sister are extremely subservient. "Esmé isn't a bit like them," he boasts. "She can speak for herself."

After several months, the doctor included Sanford in a weekly therapy group. At first, Sanford was silent. But soon he began verbally lashing out, not only at the doctor, but also at the three other males. In his individual sessions, he and the doctor discussed whether Sanford's venom was connected to ancient feelings of frustration and self-doubt caused by a male parent who had made impossible demands on him, and a male sibling who, after outdoing him, had belittled or ignored him.

For a time, Sanford's heartbeats became normal. Then they acted up again. In a dramatic session in which a lot of Kleenex was used, he admitted to the fear that his growing devotion to the doctor might indicate some hidden homosexuality.

The doctor explained that everyone is likely to become devoted to a member of the same sex as well as of the opposite sex—and that, especially in therapy, people go through a stage of unconsciously transferring old feelings toward authority figures—love, hate, sexual attraction, or fear—onto the doctor. Most patients, moreover, feel worse before they feel better. The doctor suggested Sanford begin jogging. At first Sanford complained that his heart bothered him. But after a while the pain became less. His weight was down and he began to feel better. The jogging continued. So did the sessions, both individual and group.

One day Esmé phoned the doctor. Could he give *her* an appointment?

No, he said. He could not. Unless Sanford wanted her to come.

A harassed woman with a small child walks hurriedly down the street. The child begs for ice cream. Soon it asks to go to the bathroom. It complains of fatigue. It stumbles. Impatiently the woman yanks it back onto its feet. It begins to cry.

The woman is focused on getting to her destination on time. It is not that she does not care about the child. She does care, and deeply. Indeed, if harm were to come to the child, she would abandon all other concerns. If it were to die, so would she. But right now, as often in a stressful contemporary life, she has neither the time nor the patience to attend to its needs. "Later," she says.

The woman typifies ourselves, and the child our body. It keeps telling us that it is hungry or thirsty, tired or off-balance. Eventually, we do heed the acute short-term signals. But we may continue to ignore the subtle long-term ones that denote underexercise or overwork, too much or the wrong kind of food or drink, perhaps a job that daily exposes us to noxious fumes or the kind of boss or coworker who reactivates in us some outdated emotional conflict.

For Sanford, this kind of conflict centered on an unresolved relationship with his father. In many people, a buried set of conflicting emotions may affect not only the health of an organ, such as Sanford's heart, but also the health of his cells.

Far more remains to be learned than is known about cellular action, but one of the most exciting discoveries concerns a cell's *receptor areas* (of which there may be as many as ten thousand per cell). Some receptors are aroused by different chemicals floating by in the mildly salty soup that bathes the cells inside our bodies. Each receptor acts like a lock waiting for a particular key, or like a tiny mouth that purses or widens in anticipation of a specific food. In some diabetics, different from Sanford, the normal amount of insulin is produced, but for some obscure reason, the appropriate receptor areas in their cells are not "hungry" enough to take it in. So it goes by, unused.

Far smaller than the cells are the microbes, both those that normally inhabit our body and those that occasionally arrive en masse as unwelcome guests. For example, as biologist and ethologist Desmond Morris reports, "On our healthy clean skin there is an average of five million . . . friendly microbes . . . to every square centimenter. . . . If we managed to live 'germ free' of our own microbes . . . we would be less resistant to the foreign, and really vicious, microbes that we would encounter. . . . We have to pay a price for their services, for even they can get out of hand when we become unduly stressed. Some of our diseases are caused . . . by a sudden 'overcrowding' of our 'normal' microbes."*

An example of a resident "normal" microbe that only occasionally makes its presence unpleasantly felt is herpes simplex I. It may cause a fever blister when the lip is bumped, or exposed to too much sunlight, or when the person gets a cold or, as many doctors believe, is under too much stress. But the person quickly recovers.

Tragic, however, is the situation of those patients with acquired immune deficiency syndrome (AIDS), who have little or no protection against the overcrowding either by their own "normal" microbes or the "really vicious" ones from outside.

Even for people with a well-functioning immune system, too heavy a long-term strain, whether physical or emotional, interpersonal or environmental, may cause some body part or function to "give." Today there is greater recognition than formerly of the early warning signals. A stroke, for example, is likely to flag its onset an hour—or even a week—beforehand by a fleeting symptom (transient ischemic attack, or TIA), which should be reported immediately to one's doctor, since four out of five stroke victims remember having previously noted one or more of these. †
New methods of rehabilitation from stroke, such as the experimental prompt increase of oxygen, offer hope that soon a far higher percentage of stroke victims will survive without lasting damage.

In retrospect, of course, it is easier to see what action might have prevented, or at least minimized, a serious ailment. Franklin D. Roosevelt, for example, had complained of unusual fatigue that momentous summer day in Campobello. Had he gone for a nap instead of a pick-me-up swim in the icy Atlantic, he might not have been so crippled by the polio that felled him a few hours later.

Yet F.D.R. did recover, though he lost the use of his legs. He had a potent will to live and sense of purpose (IC). He also had devoted helpers, such as Eleanor Roosevelt and Louis Howe (other people). He had the financial means to avail himself of the mineral baths in Warm Springs (environments), and, by swimming, was able to strengthen his powerful shoulders (body). Though polio restricted him to a wheelchair, his IC developed a new inner density that made people want to follow him. As

*Desmond Morris, *The Naked Ape* (New York: McGraw Hill, 1967; Dell, 1984).
†TIA symptoms are listed in Appendix C.

with his cousin Theodore Roosevelt, a former victim of tuberculosis, if a spoiled young man had not fallen gravely ill, would he ever have developed the stuff of presidency?

Such questions have long been raised by biographers, but today doctors—and patients, too—are pondering them. For while too great a burden of stress endured over too long a time can adversely affect the body's wondrous self-righting mechanisms, remaining too protected from stress may lead to their stagnation. Stagnation, moreover, can be a problem not only within an individual but also within a species. The amoeba, for example, which merely detours around its sources of stress, has not evolved in billions of years.

Human beings, in contrast, are both still evolving and never wholly free from stress. Today "stress" has become something of a code word, a medical mantra intoned to explain whatever ails us. Yet the grandfather of stress research, Hans Selye, M.D., of Montreal University, flatly said, "No disease is caused by stress alone."

There are, he said, differences, both in *types* of stress and in people's ways of *coping* with them. Some people are natural "racehorses," reveling in a fast-paced life, while others are "turtles," gravitating toward tranquil activities. Sometimes a person is a racehorse during youth and a turtle later on, or vice versa. No one, said Selye, can judge as well as the individual what his or her optimal stress level is. Even the doctor may know less than the patient in this regard.

But what the doctor does know grows curiouser and curiouser. The patient's outward behavior, for example, may give no indication of how his heart and blood vessels are responding to current stress. Some outwardly excitable people remain inwardly calm and stable, while some outwardly calm people are churning within. In animals, such as rats and monkeys, two different kinds of "churning" occur, depending on the type of stress. If the stimulus is confrontation between members of two *groups*, one set of hormones (from the adrenal cortex) is increased, while if the stimulus is *individual* humiliation, another set (from the adrenal medulla) is mobilized. Either way, the long-term effect on heart and circulation may be damaging, even though the animal has remained free of "traditional" cardiovascular risk factors, such as high blood fats (serum lipids).

While statistics do indicate that certain physical habits, such as smoking or eating too much of the wrong kinds of food, often precede the onset of heart disease, there are also emotional, relational, and environmental "final straws" that can "break the camel's back." Yet the straw that breaks the back of one camel may have a wholly different effect on another camel, or on that same camel in different circumstances.

Thus, before we blame any physical ailment entirely on the body dimension, we need to know how well the righting mechanisms of the other dimensions are operating and how well the IC is coordinating the four of them. For example, if Sanford, earlier in life, had managed to come to terms with the volatile mix of unconscious feelings he was harboring toward his father (other people), his *body* might not have acted up. Fortunately his internist was one of the growing number who now recognize certain symptoms as sometimes deriving their main impetus from beyond the dimension of body alone.

The body's own righting mechanisms were described by Harvard's great physiologist Dr. Walter Cannon as striving to achieve *homeostasis.* * This continual balancing act is needed both within and between our various organs and body systems. An oversimplified way to picture this situation is to visualize someone standing on a teeter-totter (a low, one-person seesaw). If he is pushed down on one side, he will naturally, without thought, exert extra effort on the other side.

Fortunately, our righting mechanisms operate most of the time without our needing to pay them any heed. But unfortunately, on occasion, they act too unselectively or last too long. More is not always better within the body's systems, whether digestive or respiratory, skeletomuscular or genitourinary, cardiovascular or nervous, immune or endocrine.

So distinct are these systems that their respective products may be anathema to one another. If sweat from the skin drops into the eye, it burns. Yet between people, products from the same system may blend harmoniously. A transfusion of your blood may save my life.

One example of an *unselective* reaction by a bodily system is the way in which certain white cells (lymphocytes) battle a transplanted organ as if it were an unwanted invader. Unless chemically interrupted, they will cause the body to "reject" it.

An example of a reaction that *lasts too long* is the production of hyaline by a premature baby's lungs. This shiny material protects their delicate tissue from the air for which they are not yet ready, but if its production is not reduced at birth, the hyaline may itself interfere with the lung's absorption of oxygen, sometimes causing death.

Many bodily functions not only carry on without their host's giving them a thought but perform the better for being ignored. To tell oneself, "I must have a bowel movement before that long trip," may be enough to inhibit peristalsis, while a relaxed frame of mind may facilitate success. One reason why sleep is called "the best medicine"—or why meditation is likely to be restful—is that critical self-kibitzing by the conscious mind is slowed.

Homoios is Greek for "similar"; *stasis* for "position."

The maintenance of normal body temperature is an unconscious function with which mammals are born. For humans, a rise or drop of ten degrees may mean death. Fortunately, our body has a first-class thermostat. Without this inborn air-conditioning system, the heat generated by exercising the large muscles would sizzle our brain. Instead, the heated blood moves to the skin, where two and a half million glands exude perspiration. As the sweat evaporates, the skin is cooled, and this in turn cools the blood, which returns to the muscles in a homeostatically balanced manner.

When one has a fever, however, the skin is dry, and body heat mounts. This internal cooking is one form of defense against the microbes' causing the illness, and often it succeeds. Today some doctors no longer bring down the patient's fever with drugs, because the fever itself may be curative, unless it is over 102 degrees in adults. *

What is true of fever is also true of inflammation, the hurrying of white cells, extra fluid, and heat to an injured area. In certain diseases, however, the white cells overcompensate to the point of crowding out the necessary red corpuscles. In describing meningitis, for example, Dr. Lewis Thomas says, "The defense mechanism becomes itself the disease . . . while the bacteria play the role of bystander."

Other examples of a defense-mechanism overcompensation are diarrhea (the intestine's attempt to rid itself of toxic substances) and a runny nose (the mucous membrane's attempt to rid itself of irritants).

The teeter-totter, in short, can get stuck off-balance. Fortunately, from birth onward, our body's homeostatic mechanisms are extraordinarily efficient. How else, for example, would a newborn know enough to stop nursing after sufficient milk has been drunk?

Throughout life, the maintenance of normal weight is, to a large extent, the function of the appestat. This tiny part of the central brain handles feelings of hunger and satiety so as to keep the body at its original or revised "set-point," the weight to which the body naturally tends to return after pounds have recently been gained or lost. Its operation is the classic wholesome cycle: I am hungry; I eat a sensible meal with pleasure; I feel satisfied; I occupy myself and do not even think of food for several hours; then, at the next meal, I eat well but not too much. Or if on one day I do overeat, the next day I may not feel hungry.

Yet even the lucky people whose appestat (unlike Sanford's) efficiently handles weight control may find it temporarily tipped too far in either direction by real or symbolic events:

*In the old days, some syphilis patients were deliberately infected with malaria, which brings on a very high but temporary fever. The spirochete, which causes syphilis, literally could not take the heat. But then the patient was faced with the further problem of getting rid of the malaria.

- In *body*, pain or nausea from a gallstone can kill the appetite—or several drinks can unduly whet it.
- In *mind*, mention of a lemon can cause saliva to flow—or mention of a bloody accident can dry the mouth.
- In relationships with *people*, a harsh remark by a tablemate can cause the eater to push away a full plate—or conversely, in a state of nerves, to reach for a third (and not enjoyed) piece of cake.
- In relationship to *environments*, attractive decoration and lighting have long been used by restaurants to enhance diners' appetites, while some institutions (such as the military) maintain bleak dining halls, which make mealtime unnecessarily noisy and unappetizing.
- In the IC, my willpower may be strengthened by a recent compliment on how trim I look, or weakened by no perceptible reward on the scales for my recent dieting. Some crash diets, moreover, deprive the person of needed trace minerals (electrolytes) to the point where the appestat no longer registers the feeling of being satisfied: the person, therefore, may need to exert strenuous willpower to *stop* eating after *over*eating.

In the United States, obesity is a more common problem than undernourishment, despite the shocking figure of twenty million Americans who, in 1985, were found to be suffering from hunger during at least part of a given month.* With approximately thirty-four million Americans weighing at least 20 percent above their recommended weight, obesity is now believed to rival smoking and high blood pressure as a shortener of life. On the other hand—and here is an example of how snippets of health advice can catch the layperson coming and going—to worry constantly about one's own failed attempts to lose weight is itself said by some experts to be a health hazard. Fortunately, according to Dr. Wayne Calloway, a specialist in obesity at the Mayo Clinic, there are also some "healthy obese" people. These individuals have lost much, but not all, of their extra poundage and have none of the problems ordinarily associated with overweight, such as adult-onset diabetes, elevated cholesterol and blood fats, heart and gall-bladder disease, arthritis, and respiratory problems. "Even though such persons may be above the upper limit of the acceptable weight range," says Dr. Calloway, "it would make little sense to urge them to reduce their weight further."

When overweight people with a generally sturdy IC find weight loss beyond their best efforts, there may be a hereditary factor or a proclivity induced during babyhood to produce and nourish too many fat cells. Or

*"Hunger in America: The Growing Epidemic," a 1985 report by the Physician Task Force on Hunger in America, headed by J. Larry Brown of the Harvard School of Public Health.

a form of unconscious symbolism may be at work here, with food perhaps representing the parental nurturance that the individual felt deprived of as a child. Then, too, the American cultural environment with its emphasis on thinness, for reasons of fashion as well as health, causes some people to battle their appestat, which was set for a normal weight, or to confuse their appestat with unbalanced diets. (No American, it is said, can be too rich or too thin.) Starting in the 1980s, there has been an increase in the number of cases of bulimia, a pattern of food binging followed by forced vomiting (or the taking of strong laxatives), occurring mostly among young white American women. As with anorexic patients, food or the feeling of plumpness may symbolize some form of evil to be avoided at the risk even of death.

Symbolism may also be operative in the individual's response to danger, which Dr. Cannon named "fight or flight": The adrenal level rises, the blood departs from the digestive system (in order to supply the big muscles of the back and legs), and blood sugar and oxygen intake increase. Subjectively, the mouth feels dry and the heart pounds. The symptoms that brought Sanford to the hospital were typical of someone faced by a visible or invisible serious hazard.

In animals—and presumably this was also true for our early ancestors—the fight/flight response wanes soon after the disappearance of the danger. Homeostasis then achieves a return to normal balance. But in humans, especially when their problem includes symbolic elements, this waning may take too long. Days, perhaps months, after the crisis, their teetertotter has not yet returned to balance. Perhaps the person's blood pressure is still elevated, or he is plagued by nightmares. The imbalance is particularly likely to persist if, during the time of stress, he was forced to "just sit there and take it," i.e., could not physically—or perhaps verbally—work off the feelings elicited by the perceived danger. (This was the case, for instance, with Sanford's relationships to his father and brother.) As Dr. Cannon put it, "If no action succeeds the excitement, and the stress—even worry or anxiety—persists, then the bodily changes due to stress are not a preparatory safeguard, but may in themselves be profoundly upsetting to the organism as a whole."*

The current popularity of jogging may derive, in part, from its exercising of the muscles needed for "flight"; the popularity of certain encounter-group procedures, such as primal screaming or pillow pounding, may derive, in part, from their exercising of the muscles needed for "fight."

Yet even the most assiduous jogger or pillow-pounder may not thereby

*Walter B. Cannon, M.D., *The Wisdom of the Body*, New York, W. W. Norton, 1932.

"get all the poison out of his system." One type of continuing expression of it may be a symbolic malfunction of some body organ (somatization). The soldier whose comrade was blown apart "in front of his eyes" may be led off the battlefield completely blind. Physically, however, there is nothing wrong with his eyes. But he may remain incapable of sight unless doctor or drug, hypnosis or accident, forces him to relive the agonizing experience that functionally turned off his vision, and thus perhaps, at the time, saved his sanity.

Sometimes somatization is an unconscious attempt to protect not so much the self as another person. Someone makes me mad; I want to hit him; I feel pain or weakness in my arm.* The part of me that does *not* want to hurt him has won out over the part that does, but only at the expense of one of my physical functions.

At other times, somatization is an unconscious attempt to get needed attention. The body parts that doctors have found most likely to serve as a vehicle for expressing emotion are precisely those about which the common language is richest, namely, the digestive system, the heart, and the skin:

STOMACH	*HEART*
That turns my stomach	It does my heart good
I could just eat you up	It was heart-rending
I feel sick about it	It chills my heart
That makes me puke	It was heart-warming
It gets me in the gut	My heart was in my mouth
I couldn't stomach it	My heart was in my throat
I'm fed up	My heart went pitter-pat
It's been eating at me	I speak from the heart
I hate his guts	My heart stood still
My stomach turned over	She took him to her heart
You've got a lot of gall	A heart-to-heart talk
She's full of bile	He was eating his heart out
He's eaten up with envy	She was heartbroken
He scared the shit out of me	At heart he's okay
	She spoke with a heavy heart
	He had a change of heart
	Don't take it to heart
	It was a heart-wrenching decision
	My heart skipped a beat
	I don't have the heart for it

*A Norwegian study (reported by Elmer Green in *Beyond Biofeedback*) analyzed fourteen men with paralyzed right arms. Under hypnosis, every one of them revealed that he had wanted to punch his father.

SKIN

You rub me the wrong way	My skin crawled
I get the shivers	I've got you under my skin
I was touched by your letter	Sisters under the skin
That gives me goosebumps	She's sweating it out
I almost jumped out of my skin	It made my scalp tingle

JUNE: How can this list be helpful to people?

NORMAN: If they listen to what sort of expressions they use, they may catch on to some message they are unconsciously trying to communicate. Like the people who unconsciously keep referring to their target organ, the body part that is the weakest link in their particular chain.

JUNE: Do target organs run in families?

NORMAN: Sometimes. People can inherit a susceptibility, and their life stresses may activate it—or not. You have a rickety spine, and so did your mother. Other times a weakness may be congenital—present at birth, but not hereditary—like my faulty heart valve. Or it may be a physical function that the person was brought up to believe has great symbolic significance for health.

JUNE: Like what?

NORMAN: Oh, like eating three square meals a day, or logging in eight hours of sleep, or having a bowel movement every morning. Some of my patients are sure they'll get sick if they miss out on one of these, even though, in the short run, such functions don't matter all that much.

JUNE: You mean because homeostasis will see to it that in time the person will surely eat or sleep or eliminate?

NORMAN: Not only that, but it's probably good for people to fast occasionally, or spend a night quietly thinking about their life. Also, dozing can be almost as good for you as sleep.

JUNE: What about people's target organ? How much attention should they give it?

NORMAN: I think they should stop, look, and listen, and not act like the mother who kept ignoring the whining child. After all, your target organ is you. What are you trying to tell yourself? Maybe you should slow down; maybe you should speed up. Whatever adapting you then do may head off a vicious cycle.

JUNE: You mean, the way I've learned to take Bufferin and a hot bath and lie down, when my back acts up?

NORMAN: Sure. Or the way I modify my diet when my stomach or too many of my patients act up.

JUNE: But don't some *physical* target organs also engage the person's *mental* health?

NORMAN: Yes—they can even engage *other* people's mental health.

JUNE: How?

NORMAN: The way members of certain families *all* suffer from depression. One member gets a symptom, which elicits an emotional collapse in another member, which then further upsets the first member, and so forth.

JUNE: Is that kind of thing likely to be hereditary?

NORMAN: Not necessarily. The identical twin of a schizophrenic patient may *not* develop the disease. The individual often surprises us in regard to what we think of as his target organ.

JUNE: Did Sanford's case surprise you in any way?

NORMAN: Not really. He's a lot like most cases that come to the internist: He has a physical symptom whose cause is other than purely physical. Sanford might well have been sent by his internist to a cardiologist, without any resulting long-term improvement. And then to some other doctor.

JUNE: How can people tell if they're in the same boat?

NORMAN: When their symptom isn't helped by a doctor's recommendations, or keeps returning and getting worse; or when the lab and other tests are negative or show only a small abnormality; or when the doctor isn't clear about what he's trying to treat.

JUNE: What can such patients do?

NORMAN: They can ask themselves, "Why this particular ailment at this particular time?" If the body dimension doesn't offer a clue, they can try the other three. After all, Sanford's symptoms didn't appear till he came under special strain from Esmé.

JUNE: So people with a stomachache should ask not just what they ate the day before but also where they ate it and with whom?

NORMAN: Or they can discuss their symptom with a person who knows them well. Or read up on it in a family health encyclopedia. Either way, they may discover a clue worth following up.

JUNE: What if people figure their physical problem is in their head?

NORMAN: They can consult a psychotherapist or counselor and then see if their internist agrees with the diagnosis. Or their internist, like Sanford's, may recommend a psychiatrist.

JUNE: What was it the psychiatrist did for Sanford?

NORMAN: He got Sanford to go back in his feelings to the past, and improve his current care of body. Esmé had offered to postpone the wedding. So Sanford had time to decide about his job environment. He could summon IC strength and ask for a raise, or look for another job. Either way, he'd have to deal with an authority figure. Once he had relived and sorted out his mixed feelings about his real father, he presumably could deal better with whoever the father-surrogate in his life might be. Otherwise, he might unwittingly start up a vicious cycle by offending his boss, losing his job and then maybe his girl, and further undermining his physical health.

JUNE: What about people in the opposite situation from Sanford, the ones who get blamed for symptoms in their *mind* even though the cause is in their *body*?

NORMAN: That's an important problem that doctors, as well as laypersons, should pay more attention to.

IV
Mostly Mind
Introducing Mary Ellen

"This must be happening to someone else. I could not have borne it."

> Anna Akhmatova, Russian poet
> (as her husband and son were
> being led off to prison for
> political reasons)

Mary Ellen is a slim, attractive young woman who grew up in a midwestern town with four younger sisters and an older brother. From the age of three, Mary Ellen was told to "mind the baby," and the babies kept coming. Her brother, however, was never expected to help. Even when, at the age of eight, Mary Ellen had a fever that lasted more than a month, she was expected to help with the "little ones." Visitors praised Mary Ellen, but her mother took her for granted.

Her mother ran the household. Mary Ellen's father dutifully brought home his earnings. And when conflict arose between his wife and children, he sided with his wife: "Your mother knows best."

His favorite daughter was the second one, Eloise, the blond, the "doll." Only she was able to cajole him into doing something with "the girls" (i.e., his wife and daughters). In his view, girls had their own forms of activity. It would no more occur to him to take a girl to a baseball game than expect a boy to cook.

At the age of twenty-four, Mary Ellen abruptly left home. In Boston she found a job as a secretary in an insurance company. She moved in with three young women from the office. Their apartment was pleasant, but Mary Ellen complained that the others were asking her to do more than her share of the housework. Her constant reminding of how often each had performed which chore, in turn, was irritating to them.

A young man from the office asked her for a date. She was so certain that he would be disappointed if he took her out that she brushed him off. At home she became more quiet, less likely to join in the other girls' banter.

One evening a housemate got a zipper caught in the back of her dress. Without knocking she hurried into Mary Ellen's room. Mary Ellen was lying on the bed, crying. On her night table was a large bottle of aspirin, empty.

"What's the trouble?"

"Life's not worth living."

"What do you *mean?*"

Out came the story—and up came all the aspirins.

Several months before, Mary Ellen had felt a severe pain in her chest. She went to a doctor, who asked her a lot of questions and prescribed an antidepressant. She took the medicine, but the pain grew worse. Every time she visited or phoned the doctor, he suggested that she take a higher dose of the drug. By then she was dizzy, but the doctor just said that was typical of depression. And the pain became almost constant. Life under these conditions, she felt, was simply not worth living.

The housemate canceled her date and drove Mary Ellen to the hospital. The emergency-room doctor sent Mary Ellen right to the intensive-care unit. A doctor diagnosed acute pericarditis, a painful inflammation of the sac surrounding the heart.

Toward the end of Mary Ellen's long convalescence, the chief of cardiology came to see her. He said her pericardium was healed but that she should see a psychiatrist.

"You said my pain came from that long fever I had as a kid."

"That's right. You probably had rheumatic fever."

"What does a psychiatrist have to do with *that?*"

"First of all, he can help you cope with having been treated so unsuccessfully by your internist. He gave you the wrong medicine in the wrong dose. But he wasn't wrong about your being depressed."

"How do *you* know?"

"We've been watching you for weeks. You're more limp than someone your age should be. And at times, especially in the mornings, your expression is tragic."

At the psychiatrist's office, Mary Ellen sat in the chair farthest from his desk. Her large gray eyes were fixed on the floor. Her voice was so faint that he kept asking her to speak up.

She told him that the priest to whom she went for confession also asked her to speak up. Perhaps it was because she so rarely had anything to confess. She did not steal or lie or lose her temper. She did not engage in any sexual activity. Sometimes she felt so inadequate about not having a sin to confess that she invented one—and then felt guilty about having lied.

Mary Ellen brought to the doctor a mimeographed list of admonitions that had been handed out at church the previous Sunday. She had underlined this passage: *The lot of the impenitent is "everlasting and eternal punishment" and "eternal damnation."* So terrified was she about eternal damnation that instead of allowing herself to fall in love, and thus risk some form of sexual sin, she had, by dint of one excuse or another, rebuffed all overtures by men. Furthermore, she told the doctor, if a man was interested in *her*, she automatically lost respect for his judgment.

After months of improved diet and exercise, she began to get in touch with the deep resentment she had been harboring against both her parents. Bitterly, Mary Ellen railed at her mother's having robbed her of childhood's joys. "I'll never forgive her. What she took from me I can never get back."

Her rage at her father was based on his preferring her brother to the girls, and Eloise to herself. Mary Ellen had never consciously tried to compete with her younger sister; that would have been too demeaning. But she did recall one instance when she had fibbed about Eloise and gotten her into trouble.

Despite her anger at her father, Mary Ellen still yearned for his approval—and the contradictory quality of her feelings carried over into her relationship with her boss. When he was impersonal, she worried that he hated her; when he was friendly, she worried that he wanted to seduce her. Her mother had drummed into the girls, "Men want only one thing."

Mary Ellen's performance at work was erratic. Documents she prepared for her boss were full of typos. Her doctor suggested that she consider the concept of "passive aggression." This is the way some people behave, he said, when they are more angry than they realize at someone they also wish to please. Part of the dammed-up anger is likely to "leak" onto innocent third parties.

How, Mary Ellen asked, could she prevent such leakage?

The doctor said she could try to find out what had caused the anger, or symbolically work it off through exercise or another activity. Mary Ellen asked whether learning to fly a plane would be a good idea. The more she thought about it, the more she wanted to do it. The doctor said that anything she felt that enthusiastic about was worth exploring. He also said she was well enough to enter a therapy group.

In group, however, she said little. One day, Jason, a forty-year-old optometrist, reported that her passive attitude was bugging him. "Why should such a good-looking woman just sit there like a bump?"

She burst into tears.

"Oh, for God's sake," he said. "*Now* what's wrong?"

"I'm not good-looking," she wept. "My sister is. I'm the ugly one, inside and out."

Several days later she was walking to the bus that would take her to the airfield for her flying lesson. She saw Jason and crossed to the other side of the street. He followed her. "Are you still angry?"

She stopped in surprise. "Angry? I'm not angry!"

"Oh yes you are."

She turned and stamped off. Jason's laughter followed. . . .

The painful black mood called *mild depression* occurs frequently enough to be characterized as "the common cold of the psyche." As for serious (clinical) depression, the milestone 1984 census by the National Institute of Mental Health estimates that, in any six-month period, this disease will afflict 5 to 6 percent of Americans.*

As for psychosomatic ailments, the World Health Organization estimates that depression is involved in one-fifth of the world's deaths from chronic heart and gastroenteric disease.

Although prolonged depression can ultimately undermine the IC, a tendency to depression cannot be equated with a weak IC. Abraham Lincoln, for example, a man of prodigious inner resources, maturity, and wisdom, suffered intermittent attacks of severe depression. Whether or not depression will be proved to stem from a slight imbalance in the chemistry and electromagnetism of the brain, it certainly responds, sometimes dramatically, to psychotropic drugs, or to a supplement of the body's own trace mineral, lithium carbonate. Also helpful in reversing depression are individual and group psychotherapy, and, as a last resort, electroconvulsive therapy (ECT, or shock treatment). Most depressions, fortunately, seem to be self-limited, clearing up after a miserable eight months or less. In fact, as Frederick K. Goodwin, M.D., chief of research at the National Institute of Mental Health, says, "Depression is one of the mental illnesses that can be completely cured."

*The ailment that occurs with greatest frequency is *anxiety disorder* (which includes phobias, panic states, and obsessive-compulsive disorders). Second are the disorders of substance abuse; third are the affective disorders that include depression. The overall estimate is that over a six-month period, one-fifth of all Americans are affected by some mental disorder(s). And only a fifth of them receive psychiatric treatment.

Some depressions are called "situational," meaning that they are trig-gered by the environment—something social or economic, for instance. Maggie Scarf, author of *Unfinished Business: Pressure Points in the Lives of Women*, describes a cross-current of values that has been precipitating depression in many American women, especially young and middle-aged ones. "Establish your identity by way of an ongoing career" is one message; "Have your babies early in life for the sake of their health" is another. On the one hand, women are told, "Success is what matters," and on the other, "Intimacy is what counts." Not only are many women confused about what they should do, but their body may be pulling them in one direction while their mind (or career) is pulling in another.

Why does one person succumb to depression or other mental ills, and another person not? Why does the depressed person succumb at one time of life and not another? Causes include genetic predisposition, society's lack of appreciation for that individual's mix of talents, and the brain's incapacity to produce enough of certain chemicals nicknamed the "neu-rojuices."

Perhaps the most exciting field of all current research is neurology, especially the branch studying the brain. Two opposite approaches are bringing results. One is to map the incredibly complex operations of the brain as a whole—as a system. The other is to identify what the different sections of the brain are doing. Already mapped are some tiny specific areas where vivid memories of sight and sound can be elicited. Also mapped are areas where diseases such as Parkinson's and Alzheimer's may someday be reversed by implants of cells that make up for shortages of crucial neurojuices.

Through use of Positron Emission Transaxial Tomography (the PETT scanner), researchers are able to inject a radioactive sugarlike tracer into the bloodstream and then spot which brain sections utilize it most under which type of circumstance. Such experiments have shown that demen-tia, Huntington's chorea, depression, epilepsy, and stroke, each affect brain function in a different way. At the same time, anatomical and biochemical differences are showing up between the brains of autistic and schizophrenic patients and those of other people.

An example of the whole-brain approach is the work of Roger Sperry, M.D., professor of psychobiology at the California Institute of Tech-nology. His focus of attention is itself a mind-twister, namely, as he puts it, how "conscious effects work *into* brain activity as well as being derived *from* it." Someday, perhaps, this kind of circular interaction may provide a key to operations by the IC itself.

Unusual is the way that the human brain differs from much of the rest of the universe which is running down or disintegrating (entropy). Instead, the brain's evolutionary hallmark is an ever greater degree of energy becoming ever better integrated.

So energetic is the brain that it uses 70 percent of the sugars we ingest, and 20 percent of the oxygen we inhale, although it represents only 2 percent of our total body weight.

The brain, furthermore, though intimately connected with the body, is also separated from it by the "blood-brain barrier." This barrier acts like a combination of customs official and export-control officer. Its mission is to keep *out* the chemicals that the brain does not want, and keep *in* those that the brain cannot afford to share.

Avocado-textured and gray, our brain is the most intricate three-pound unit yet discovered anywhere. It is composed of a hundred billion nerve cells, each of which has a thousand possible connections with other cells. *

In the course of evolution, Lyall Watson, author of *Lifetide*, suggests, when the human brain reached around seven hundred cubic centimeters—the size, say, of a cantaloupe—what is called consciousness first arose.† Remains and relics, such as those of Cro-Magnon man in the caves of France, reveal that early Homo sapiens had a large brain and stunning artistic achievement. Says Watson, "A critical size was reached where a small quantitative increase in brain substance resulted in a dramatic qualitative change in function."

Today, the average brain occupies fourteen hundred cubic centimeters, though some people own one as large as two thousand or as small as one thousand without being more or less bright than their neighbors. Unfortunately, the large size of the human brain, together with its protective encasement in bone, makes for a difficult trip down the birth canal. From the vantage point of the individual's mental health, he might have done better to remain for longer than nine months in the womb; but from the vantage point of the mother's physical health, this would have been impossible.

According to Paul McLean, M.D., of the National Institutes of Health, the human brain has evolved in three anatomically and chemically dis-

---

*The economist Kenneth Boulding, past president of the American Association for the Advancement of Science, once estimated that even if each of the brain's neurons were capable of only two states—namely, on or off—their capacity would be 2^{10} billionth power. (Actually brain neurons are now recognized as capable of *more* than two states.) To write out this number, says Dr. Boulding, at the rate of one digit per second, would take ninety years. In comparison, the number of neutrinos (smaller even than atoms) that could be packed into the universe could be written in only four minutes.

†Lyall Watson, *Lifetide: The Biology of the Unconscious*, New York: Simon and Schuster, 1979.

tinct parts, each of which continues to fulfill an essential function. His shorthand for the three are our *reptile*, *mammal*, and *primate* brains.

Deepest down is the subcortex, or "reptile brain," which handles the involuntary reflexes that control gland function and body growth, heart action and blood-vessel expansion and contraction, digestion and sleep. Here, presumably, lies what Dr. Walter B. Cannon termed "the wisdom of the body." Yet far more than simple homeostasis goes on. The typical reptile in McLean's laboratory, for example, assumes symbolic postures by instinct and adapts to the behavior of the group by imitation.*

Lizards, on arising, first seek out the warmth of the sun (or its laboratory equivalent), for they lack homeostatic heat control. Later they venture forth, find breakfast, have a bowel movement, greet their friends, ritually show off for members of the opposite—or their own—sex, enjoy a spot of lunch, go home for a nap, and return for more posturings. Dr. McLean has remarked that some committee meetings remind him of his lizards.

Surrounding our "reptile brain," like a hand held over a fist, is the "mammal brain" (or midbrain), which handles activities essential to the survival of the individual and the species. These include hunting in a band, battling an enemy, and protecting one's young (lizards have zero interest in their offspring). Sometimes the needs of individual and species conflict; sometimes they coincide. An example of their conflicting is when a male chimpanzee drops back from the fleeing troop in order to battle the predator and enable the females and youngsters to escape. An example of their coinciding is the act of nursing: the enthusiastic offer of the mother's full breast to the baby's hunger, thus helping him to survive and herself to be more comfortable.

Atop the "mammal brain" is the "primate brain," the cerebral cortex. This section comprises 85 percent of the human brain and is divided into two hemispheres. Here is the biological basis for the expression "on the one hand . . . and on the other." The left lobe (which in most people controls the right side of the body) is the verbal one, where ideas march in logical sequence, where time is more significant than space, where arithmetic is learned. The right lobe, generally controlling the left side of the body, is where patterns, concepts, spatial forms (such as the human face) are apprehended, where music and painting are appreciated, and creative insights arise. The adage "The left hand is the dreamer" reflects common recognition of the imaginative power of the "right brain."

The distinctive qualities of each lobe are highlighted when accident,

---

*The first appointment Norman and June had to visit McLean at his lab was canceled by his secretary, who announced, "The lizards will be out of town; they're going to a scientific meeting."

injury, or surgery (as for intractable epilepsy) severs the corpus callosum, the two-hundred-million-fiber network that links the two hemispheres. Then, literally, "the right hand does not know what the left hand is doing." One of these "split-brain" patients, for example, kept pulling his pants down with one hand while pulling them up with the other.

Under stress, human beings often unconsciously return (regress) to an earlier developmental stage. This return may be personal, as in crying over minor frustrations as did the baby all of us once were. It may also be evolutionary, as in the hospital patient's exclusive concentration on the simplest digestive functions, in a manner reminiscent of the reptile. Regression at a personal level is useful in psychotherapy. At an evolutionary level it is useful during interludes such as childbirth, when many a woman with no conscious inkling of what to do has tapped into her mammal brain for guidance that seemed miraculous ("How did my body get so smart?").

The other side of the story is the fatigue that sometimes besets everyone's IC after a hard day of trying to coordinate the three evolutionary sections of the brain, the two lobes of the cerebral cortex, and the millions of interacting bodily subsections and *their* subsections.

The late Dr. Wilder Penfield, professor of neurosurgery at McGill University, made medical history when he first caused conscious patients, with brain exposed, to experience either dramatic visions or melodic sounds, feelings of murderous rage or ineffable bliss, depending on which tiny area he was stimulating with an electrode. Future charting of pleasure centers in the brain may point to ways in which an unhealthful habit, such as drug addiction or smoking, can be overcome. A rat with an implanted microelectrode in one of his pleasure centers will both ignore food to the point of starvation (death of the individual) and also abstain from available sex (death to the species). In humans, perhaps, when the appestat area of the brain is better mapped and subject to corrective stimulation, people will no longer want to eat or drink more than is good for them.

José Delgado, M.D., then at the Yale Medical School, used electrodes in a bull's brain to make him charge—and, at other times, turn into a gentle Ferdinand—at the doctor's will, by way of radio control. Dr. Delgado has also caused human patients to form a fist and turn their heads by sending current through appropriately placed electrodes in their brains. Subjectively, the patients were convinced that their actions were voluntary.

For the patient troubled by chronic pain or involuntary movement of his muscles, Drs. Irving Cooper of Westchester (N.Y.) County Medical Center and Robert Fischell of Johns Hopkins Applied Physics Laboratory have implanted a rechargeable "neuropacemaker" that the patient can use to relieve both conditions. Other innovators foresee a comparable stimulator of neurotransmitters through an implanted pump that could deliver these chemicals to the brain.

Contrary to what one would assume, the connections *inside* a brain cell are electrical, while *between* cells (across the synapse) the connections are chemical. More of the brain's circulating chemicals are being identified all the time, and the complexity of their interactions is enough to boggle the mind. The same brain cell, for example, may have receptor areas for both a specific neurochemical *and its antagonist.* "If the brain were so simple that we could understand it," writes G. Edgin Pugh, author of *The Biological Origin of Human Values,* "we would be so simple that we couldn't."*

One matter on which all brain researchers agree is that neurotransmitters do not act in isolation. Their interaction, however, is incredibly difficult to track because their rapidity is so great and their amounts are so small. For example, the quantity of a particular hormone that a relatively uncomplicated body cell can pick up has been compared to a pinch of salt in Walden Pond.

Tiny amounts of brain serotonin, one of the neurojuices, are now thought to protect people from the subjective anguish that leads to suicide. Dr. Frederick K. Goodwin and his associates at the National Institute of Mental Health studied a group of young mental patients over many years. The patients who eventually killed themselves turned out to have had a lower-than-average level of brain serotonin in their urine. During their lifetimes, moreover, they had also demonstrated a higher-than-average level of aggression. Thus Freud's hypothesis, that brain chemistry is involved in serious mental illness, is being borne out. † Some unsuccessful attempts at suicide, however, such as Mary Ellen's swallowing a bottleful of aspirin tablets, are viewed less as a determination to die than as a wordless plea for help. Other suidical acts, successful as well as failed, appear as attempts to punish someone else (the "secondary victim") as well as the self. A propensity to suicide, like that toward alcohol abuse, keeps recurring in some families, giving rise to the conjecture that a hereditary tendency may be involved.

Recent studies of alcoholics have shown, in addition to considerable

*G. Edgin Pugh, *The Biological Origin of Human Values,* (New York: Basic Books, 1977).

†Other studies suggest that the violent behavior of some criminals is also accompanied by unusually low levels of brain serotonin. At the same time, unusually high levels of epinephrin may inhibit action by the immune system. So, again, more is not always better.

brain-cell death, some physiological changes in the *structure* and *composition* of the membranes surrounding those cells that dictate emotions, memory, and most bodily functions. In autopsies of mental patients who suffered nightmarish hallucinations, the *position* of certain brain cells appears to have been a factor in their painful symptom.

Important research is now focusing on the individual brain cells and their "appetites." Cells typically refuse to accept the chemical appropriate to their receptor areas if a similar chemical has recently preceded it. This form of cell action might be compared to a lock that is jammed with chewing gum and therefore will not respond to its key. When a heroin addict gets a shot of nalaxone, an opiate-antagonist, his subsequently injected heroin (an opiate) will have none of its usual effect. On the other hand, some cells develop over time an apparent allergy to specific chemicals so that even a trace of one will inflame their receptor areas.

To use a brain cell as analogy to the personality as a whole, it is possible that a person, because of some past unresolved conflict, may unconsciously develop emotional "receptor areas" that are overly sensitive to later versions of this conflict. The person, therefore, may find himself violently overreacting, yet, like Sanford and Mary Ellen, not be consciously aware of what he is reacting against.

That there may be a *physical* basis for such vulnerability is indicated by recent research. According to neuroscientist Jonathan Winson of New York City's Rockefeller University, early childhood includes a "critical period" during which the cerebral cortex is developing: "Once this period passes, that brain circuitry will not easily change; the unconscious is captured in this circuitry and its many connections to the brain's emotional center, the limbic system."*

While experiences that have been *sup*pressed are more or less subject to voluntary recall, those that were dynamically *re*pressed into the deep unconscious are not. Perceived at the time as too threatening, they have, so to speak, been relegated to the ship's hold, where they remain like hungry dogs in a cage, growling and straining. Much of a person's energy may unconsciously be diverted into keeping them in place. †

When a big wave from outside strikes the ship of self, or when a heavy emotional burden is taken aboard, some of the dogs may spring loose. The person may need help in recaging them or, better yet, in retraining them so that they can wander free. For what was once feared by a small

*Daniel Goleman, "Is Analysis Testable As Science, After All?" *New York Times*, 22 January 1985.
†In modern psychiatric parlance, the term *unconscious* has supplanted *subconscious* because it does not carry the same connotation of being inferior to conscious thought.

child as a slavering mastiff may, when that person is grown, seem no more vicious than a cocker spaniel.

Children who cannot face the hatred they felt when frustrated by a loved parent or sibling may, for example, repress the whole episode. The buried rage entangled with love may thereafter emerge only in symbolic form. The person may, like Sanford, express his semimurderous feelings while driving a car, or, like Mary Ellen, turn the unrecognized hatred in against the self. "Depression," said Freud, "is the underbelly of anger." Or the person may use passive aggression, as Mary Ellen did, or explode in otherwise inexplicable violence (such as abuse of a child, parent, or spouse). Or the person may not register anger against anyone, no matter how valid the provocation ("I am one of those people who never get mad"). For some people, a prolonged "swallowing" of their rage may augment throat or stomach problems. As Cambridge, Massachusetts, psychiatrist Leston Havens says, "The extent of murderousness in the whole human race is not readily acknowledged despite the facts of widespread war, homicide, and suicide."

On the other hand, a person without a repressed dark side might grow up without the coiled energy necessary to pursue a long-term skill or purpose. If surgeons had no dynamically buried hostility, they might not enjoy the creative cutting of patients; if psychiatrists had no dynamically buried curiosity about sex, as psychiatrist Fritz Redlich cheerfully suggests, they might not enjoy creatively probing other people's secrets. Or if theater buffs—and fans of books, movies, and TV—had no dynamically buried destructiveness, they might not enjoy the catastrophes suffered by the characters on page or stage. Nor is it an accident that the Greek tragedians, along with Shakespeare, repeatedly dealt with the most forbidden of impulses: incest with parent, sibling, or offspring; murderous rivalry with blood relative or mate; betrayal of God or country to save the self or loved one(s). Their audiences still emerge exhausted but somehow at peace. What Aristotle termed the "proper purgation of the emotions," Freud called the "unconscious defense of sublimation."

Though what is repressed is not directly accessible to its owner's consciousness, indirectly it may make its presence known through the clues it leaves. Such clues, Freud demonstrated, often include otherwise insignificant events, like misspeaking or being late. If I never allow myself to be pleased by someone, I may unconsciously be trying to exert control over him, or even over another person whom he symbolically represents. One of the simpler definitions of mental health is "the ability to live fully in the present" (i.e., not remain obsessed with old repressions). Another is the willingness to be pleased, some of the time, by some of the people, including oneself.

The principles by which the deep unconscious operates are not the same as those of the conscious mind. Yet sometimes they can be identified by the conscious mind. Moreover, if, like Rumpelstiltskin, one can call them by name, they may lose much of their power to hurt. These principles include the following:

- Time has no meaning. In the realm of repression, there is no calendar. What one felt as an infant may be felt with equal acuteness by an adult.
- Space has no meaning. As in dreams, one can be in two places at once. A by-product is that there is nowhere to hide.
- Linear logic or consistency has no meaning. I may both passionately want to hurt someone and also desperately fear lest harm come to him.
- There is magic thinking: If I wish hard enough, I can cure someone's terminal illness—or conversely, by wishing hard enough, I can cause him to wither and die. There is a blurring, thus, between wish and deed. If, while I am angry at him, he should fall ill, I may unconsciously fear that it was my anger that caused the illness—and I may suffer inappropriate guilt that is unassuageable by logic.
- Tit-for-tat or "an eye for an eye" is the expected form of human exchange. If I fear that my anger caused someone's illness, I may further fear that he, in retaliation, will cause me to fall ill. Thus, added to my guilt may be a further burden of fear. Or, fearing his retaliation, I may unconsciously head it off by injuring myself. Propitiatory self-harm may be an attempted return to the helplessness of infancy, which tends to arouse the protective, rather than punitive, impulse in adults.
- Outdated patterns may continue to dominate a person's life. At a time of high fever, for example, I may crave milk, as in infancy, even though milk, like other protein, is proscribed during fever, and the body, if left to itself, would probably have the "wisdom" to spurn it.
- Unconscious conflicts are likely to appear in symbolic disguise. In the deep unconscious—as in remembered dreams—one's emotions, like children playing with a trunk full of costumes, make their appearance as something else. "The dream," said Freud, "is the royal road to the unconscious." The dream is also a necessity for long-term sanity. During experiments, people who were awakened several nights in a row when they started dreaming became disoriented, depressed, even subject to dreamlike hallucinations while awake. "The symbolizing impulse," says Dr. Robert J. Lifton, author of *The Broken Connection*, "is no less elemental than the death-terror." Without that symbolizing impulse, human culture, like individual dreams, would be much the poorer.

Dreams, like the arts, provide us with a valuable safety-valve. Feared events may be rehearsed, forbidden acts relished. Memories, like dice, may be shaken up and thrown again, relationships revised. While a dream's symbolism may appear to the waking mind as primitive in the sense of unsophisticated, it may also be primitive in the sense of touching base with the oldest, most fundamental parts of the brain.

Freud stressed the importance of symbolic disguise at the individual level; Carl Jung stressed it at the collective level. According to Jung, an individual is affected not only by the personal contents of his own unconscious, but also by the general patterns of the "collective unconscious." Some of these patterns comprise what he termed *archetypes*. Here loom the primal figures of fairy tale and myth, the king-father and earth-mother, the special child and priest-healer, the demon-destroyer (male and female) and rescuing angel (female and male).

Archetypes are not only significant in the rituals of all documented cultures but also vividly experienced at the family level by the small child. To the infant, parents are believed to appear not as the well-meaning but fallible adults that in fact they are, but as awesome ogres or angels, omnipotent and omniscient, from whom the most secret childish yearnings could not possibly be hidden.

Within the child's immature brain, the parent is also likely to be viewed not as in a smoothly flowing motion picture, but in one that suddenly stops—with a particular freeze-frame symbolizing for that child, perhaps for life, the essence of that adult. The frame may reveal a moment that was insignificant from the adult's point of view, perhaps a reaction not even focused on the child. For Sanford, for example, the freeze-frame of scowl lines between his father's eyes implied paternal disapproval of Sanford, while in reality they represented a complexion weatherbeaten from years at sea. For Mary Ellen the freeze-frame was of her father's indulgent smile directed not, alas, at herself but, rather, at three-year-old Eloise tripping in, wearing her mother's high heels. (As playwright Arthur Miller once said, no two siblings ever have the same parent.) Whatever the mood of the freeze-frame, it may come to symbolize for life the child's relationship to that adult—or perhaps to all persons of that gender, even all human beings.

The first "transference," therefore, is that of a baby unconsciously imbuing the mother-figure or father-figure with horns or halo appropriate to a collective, superhuman or subhuman, archetype. Contrary to many people's assumption, a patient's transference onto his psychiatrist is a subsequent one—though doubtless related to the first.

It was Freud who spotted the significance of transference. For years he had been puzzled, even annoyed, by patients, especially female ones, who developed all kinds of passionate emotions toward him. He had, moreover, done nothing except sit behind the couch to elicit this mixed love and hate, trust and terror. Yet once he recognized the significance of the transferred feelings, he refused to terminate treatment until after the patient had relived them and learned to redirect their energy into more appropriate, wholesome, and satisfying channels.

An unconscious effort to lessen emotional pain is what triggers the mind's righting mechanisms. These "unconscious defenses" are used daily by everyone. In manageable form, they fend off the realization of what might be intolerable, or even too distracting, if fully faced at that moment. In extreme form, they are used by mentally ill people to diminish contact with what others call reality.

One of the most frequently used defenses is *denial*. A self-strengthening example appears at the opening of this chapter, when Anna Akhmatova refused to take in the total anguish involved in the arrest of her husband and son. A self-weakening example is that of the man who does push-ups in the course of a suspected heart attack just to prove that he is not having one.

The unconscious defenses are described by Harvard psychiatrist George Vaillant as "psychological white corpuscles."* As with their physical counterparts, in the right amounts, they are essential to preserve and regain good health, but "too much of a good thing" may constitute a health hazard. Vaillant further believes that identifying these defenses was Freud's most valuable discovery.

The two defenses that American society seems most often to reward are *sublimation* and *humor*. Yet these—like denial— can be overdone. An example of sublimation overdone was Thomas Merton's choice to live in a monastery that imposed such severe vocational deprivations that he repeatedly fell ill, physically and emotionally. An example of humor overdone caused Cervantes to observe, "It is ill joking of death in the house of a man who was hanged." Humor's tie-in with people's repressed components is revealed by the explosive quality of the laughter that greets an off-color or hostility-laden joke. If the punchline needs explaining, thus involving the listener's conscious mind, there is no comparable eruption of banked-down emotion.

The defenses, being unconscious, work much like physical homeostasis: They switch on automatically, rather than selectively, and may outlast their usefulness. At such times, a comment by friend, relative, or doctor may reveal that the person being most fooled by the defenses is their host.

In addition to sublimation, humor, and denial, other frequently used defenses include:

*George Vaillant, *Adaptation to Life* (Boston: Little, Brown, 1977).

- Projection: Not realizing how angry I am at someone, I begin worrying that he is angry with me.*
- Displacement: Not realizing how angry I am at my spouse, I yell at the dog.
- Rationalization: A fat woman squeezing into her too-tight dress insists that it must have shrunk at the cleaners.
- Intellectualization: When told I have cancer, I am so busy reading up on each type of it that whenever my friend phones, I have a new fact for him. The intellecutal activity that masks my fear, however, may also prevent me from registering his warmth and attentiveness.
- Reaction-formation: "I *love* baby," the toddler may insist, but wise parents keep a watchful eye lest toddler's "love pat" knock baby off the couch. Similarly, if a man marries a woman who seems the exact opposite of his mother, he may still be as maternally attached as the man who married his mother's clone.

Whatever someone's defenses may be, they should generally not be challenged unless the challenger has time and patience, affection and willingness to share responsibility for the consequences. New York psychoanalyst Joel S. Kovel, M.D., warns professionals as well as laypersons against moving too fast in this realm: "Harm in therapy usually occurs as a result of a too-rapid dissipation of defenses against deep anxieties."

To get in touch with the deep unconscious, Freud and his followers used verbal techniques, such as free association, analysis of dreams and slips of the tongue. Today, psychotherapists frequently make use of non-verbal techniques as well. These include Gestalt, bioenergetic exercises, Rolfing, and deep massage. One theory about such activities is that they give access to memory-traces (called *engrams*) formed in earliest babyhood, before speech had developed and when, to the not-yet-fully-formed brain, the world appeared as a confusing, unpredictable, and terrifying place. So threatening, in fact, may this infantile experience have been that it was thoroughly repressed and remains unavailable to recall through use of words.

All of us may retain emotional vestiges of our earliest months, when we were incapable of distinguishing essential boundaries, such as between self and mother, mouth and breast. Infants are also at a loss to comprehend that a parent who steps away from the cribside is not gone forever. Yet even the most devoted parent cannot be at the cribside twenty-four hours a day.

*A complex political example was Martin Luther King, Jr.'s suggestion that well-meaning whites were projecting their guilty anger onto blacks and then feeling fearful of these blacks.

It may, therefore, be that the "reservoir of ill will" with which many humans reach adolescence or young adulthood derives in part from unavoidable insecurities based on having been born with so undeveloped a brain that the IC has only primitive capacities to work with. The feelings assumed to accompany the insecurities of infancy include primal terror of desertion ("separation anxiety"), paroxysmal rage at not getting what one wants when one wants it, insatiable demand for overt affection, and unbearable conflict over remaining dependent for this affection—indeed, for life itself—on the very person(s) likely to be the focus of the terror, the rage, and the insatiability.

Different individuals at different stages respond in different ways to profound inner conflict. Fight and flight are two classic responses; one can rage at others or inwardly withdraw. But a third defense also exists—namely, to lie low. This unconscious slowing of life forces may be related to the hibernation urge in animals. It may also explain some otherwise puzzling symptoms, such as those of depression. In his book *When I Say No I Feel Guilty*, Manuel Jo Smith asserts: "Although depression would appear to have little . . . survival value today, its worth to our ancestors becomes clear if we look at how you or I behave when we become depressed. In fact, we hardly behave at all. . . . Our ancestors who got depressed and just sat around during very frustrating times . . . increased their chances of survival until better times came along."*

JUNE: Would it have helped Mary Ellen to be told her depression was like hibernation? Or that she was projecting her feelings toward her father onto her boss?

NORMAN: Not right away. The patient needs first to develop trust in the doctor. Then she needs to build up confidence that the doctor will be strong enough to support her when she summons the nerve to let go of some important unconscious defense.

JUNE: Why?

NORMAN: So much painful anxiety may be released.

JUNE: Is that the reason people should beware of irresponsible encounter groups?

NORMAN: One of many. Another is that the group may treat one of its vulnerable members as a scapegoat.

JUNE: But people have to do *something* when they're depressed!

*Manuel Jo Smith, *When I Say No I Feel Guilty* (New York: Bantam, 1975).

NORMAN: They do. They should visit a doctor skilled in the use of the many effective new drugs. Mary Ellen's first doctor was unaware of how ignorant he was in this field.

JUNE: What if a person's depression isn't that serious?

NORMAN: Well, one thing would be to try out some new activity in each dimension.

JUNE: Like what?

NORMAN: Oh, rearrange your furniture, or eat at an unfamiliar restaurant (environments), see a good friend you haven't seen in a long time (other people), take a brisk walk (body), or try to articulate what's bothering you (mind). In one way or another, your IC may act like a kaleidoscope in letting you see your problem in a new context or pattern.

JUNE: How can laypeople tell when they're overusing one of their defenses?

NORMAN: When a self-defeating pattern keeps recurring in their behavior.

JUNE: Like always apologizing?

NORMAN: Sure. I had a tennis partner who kept apologizing for every shot. I asked her to quit it—and she played much better.

JUNE: If people decide to free themselves from some unconscious defense, how should they go about it?

NORMAN: Ask for feedback from friends. Good friends are the best form of health insurance. Jason, the fellow in Mary Ellen's therapy group, ended up helping her a lot.

JUNE: But sometimes friends say things that hurt.

NORMAN: Then ask a second friend for his opinion of that comment. If the second one thinks the remark was unfair, then the first one, like Mary Ellen, may be harboring unrecognized envy.

JUNE: Poor Mary Ellen. I think envy is the *worst* thing to feel.

NORMAN: But it's part of the human condition. Our emotions are built in.

JUNE: Why should envy be built in?

NORMAN: Maybe to stimulate us to imitate what works for other people. Anyway, it's better to recognize that an emotion is part of our constitution than try to push it out of our consciousness.

JUNE: What can people do about an emotion in themselves that they hate?

NORMAN: They can "own it," that is, accept the fact that they feel it, instead of trying to deny its existence even to themselves.

JUNE: Can people neutralize a distasteful emotion, like jealousy?

NORMAN: Sure. They can, for example, force themselves to think in very specific terms. If they're jealous of someone for having a Cadillac, they should picture in detail how hard it is to park.

JUNE: Sort of a purposeful "sour grapes"?

NORMAN: Yes, but very detailed. If they envy someone for his money, they should think of all the accountants and lawyers he has to deal with.

JUNE: What should Mary Ellen have done?

NORMAN: She could have faced the fact that, sure, her brother was lucky enough to be a male; and sure, her sister was lucky enough to be pretty; but she, Mary Ellen, had a lot of qualities worth developing.

JUNE: And that her particular combo of qualities was unique?

NORMAN: What you call "combo" is part of the IC. If Mary Ellen had rallied her IC, she might have felt up to the effort of *accepting* love.

JUNE: Why should that take effort?

NORMAN: It makes us vulnerable to the person who loves us. It is hard to overestimate the effect that other people, individually and together, have on our total health.

V
Mostly Relationships With Other People

Introducing Dorothy

> "An entire generation has been raised to believe that dieting, exercise, inoculations, and other forms of preventive care are the means to avoid disease and premature death. The idea that another crucial element . . . is the ability to maintain human relationships seems strangely 'unscientific.' Yet . . . loneliness and isolation can literally 'break your heart.' "
>
> —James J. Lynch, The Broken Heart

Dorothy is the only child of Martha and Peter who are divorced. She is in her late twenties, with beautiful blond hair and a fine complexion, but she weighs two hundred pounds. Though she and George have been married five years, she claims he has never understood her; and she doesn't understand why he can't—or won't—keep a job for more than six months. Fortunately, she has steady work as an obstetrical nurse.

When Dorothy awakens in the morning, she can scarcely get out of bed. She figures that a big breakfast will provide needed energy. It does—for about an hour. Though she is a fast eater, she is usually late for work. Her knees and feet hurt (as do those of many overweight people). At her coffee break, she has a candy bar for a pick-me-up. By afternoon she is yawning. She often leaves work early, complaining about digestive problems.

The nurses on her station resent her shaving her work time, and she senses their resentment; but she cannot persuade herself to stay. As for her patients, she enjoys witnessing the birth of the infants but has little sympathy when the mother's labor is difficult.

When George gets home, he often finds Dorothy too tired to cook, so they go to a restaurant. He likes a long cocktail hour. When they get home, Dorothy is too sleepy to make love. She falls asleep at 10:00, but at 2:00 A.M. is wide awake and thirsty. She worries that if she does not get her full eight hours, she will be draggier than usual at work. She takes a sleeping pill. Too soon the alarm is buzzing. With her large breakfast, she drinks two extra cups of coffee. Later her hands tremble and she quarrels with a fellow nurse.

Dorothy's relationship with her mother, Martha, was based on a sense of duty. They never fought, but neither did they share anything important. Dorothy also dutifully visits her father, Peter, every few months. Their conversation remains superficial, except when he instructs her to lose weight. He thinks that anything connected with childbirth is disgusting, so she cannot discuss her job with him.

Is Dorothy sick? Certainly she does not feel well. But her internist can locate no evidence for diabetes, low thyroid, or other hormonal problem. In a scolding tone reminiscent of her father's, he tells her to lose weight. On her way home she is so dispirited that she treats herself to a double-chocolate ice-cream cone: "I deserve *some* pleasure."

Dorothy feels cheated by life. To compensate, she denies herself nothing that goes in the mouth. Yet after overeating, she despises herself—and that makes her defensive toward other people. George has long since given up disagreeing openly with her. The more isolated Dorothy feels, the more likely she is to console herself with food. The more bloated she becomes, the more edgy she is with people. . . .

One day Dorothy's supervisor reported to her the many complaints coming from nurses and patients. If Dorothy wanted to keep her job, she would have to consult a psychiatrist.

Though Dorothy was furious, she had little choice. She started treatment with a woman recommended by the hospital, but months went by before she developed enough trust in the doctor to make a real effort.

After half a year she began losing weight. She was elated! But soon she became extremely anxious, and the anxiety expressed itself through casting blame onto other people. Although the therapist had given her a reduced fee, Dorothy accused her of overcharging, of not allotting the full forty-five minutes, of not paying enough attention to what she said, of yawning too often, of making excuses for George or the supervisor or whoever else Dorothy had accused of being "incredibly rude."

Dorothy started stealing small items out of stores: "They rip people off anyway." She had two minor but jarring car accidents and insisted they were both the other driver's fault.

When the therapist went on vacation, Dorothy panicked. Several phone sessions were necessary. Even so, she gained a lot of weight. But after the doctor returned, Dorothy returned to her diet. Because the diet excluded alcohol, George began drinking more with his male friends and getting home later and later. The later he was, the hungrier and angrier she would be. Then he lost his job. Dorothy asked if he would come with her to the psychiatrist. He refused. They had some bitter, searing fights. One night in a rainstorm, his speeding car skidded into a tree. He was dead on arrival at the hospital.

Dorothy went into shock. Later she railed at the psychiatrist for not having forced George to visit. She also blamed the doctor for not taking better care of *her*. "Look at me," she said. "I'm hardly any thinner than when I started."

After several months of not paying her bill, she announced she was not returning and would not pay what she owed. She departed.

Within a year, however, the doctor received a phone call about her from a nearby hospital. . . .

In terms of relationship to one's fellows, humankind stands somewhere between the bee and the amoeba.

Amoebas do not need one another at all, ever. Their manner of reproducing is to divide down the middle, with each side wending its separate way, growing to full size, and dividing again.

Bees, like ants, need each other night and day, year in and out. A Thoreau is unknown in the bee world. Within the hive, the functions of daily living are carried out by different groups that are each genetically programmed to perform precisely their one task. Generalists have no place. Indeed, if a bee is prevented from doing its *own* thing, it cannot, in effect, do anything. Bees' dependence on one another is inborn and inescapable. Workers work; breeders breed; fighters fight; drones drone; and the queen queens it over the others. Their system is closed and rigidly hierarchical.

Humans, on the other hand, are remarkably adaptable, and although hierarchies keep being established both within and between their societies, these are not, as history shows, inexorably fixed.

What *is* inexorably fixed is the need of one human being for another. As psychiatrist Willard Gaylin states in his book, *Caring*, "Man is not, technically speaking, an individual. Man is an obligate social animal; a social structure is part of his biology and a necessary part of his functioning. We are a social animal not by election but by nature." Individuals, he adds, need each other not only as individuals, but also as fellow members of a group: "The group itself is a genetic fact of man's nature and the assurances for group-survival are part of the protoplasmic component of each individual member of the group."*

Some societies—Japan is a notable example—stress this group dimension more than does the individualistic U.S.A. So do many Africans. Through their frequent rituals, they celebrate man as *Homo communalis* and *Homo festivus* (as well as *Homo fantasia*, the maker of symbols), whereas in the industrialized West man seems valued primarily as *Homo sapiens*.†

As for one-to-one relationships, the first of these occurs between fetus and mother. If she should die, so most likely would the fetus (though, in all probability, she could survive its death). At the same time, the fetus already has its own potential character-print. The particular genes that happened to converge when that ovum was fertilized by that sperm have caused the fetus to be unique, all the way from the protein configurations of its cells to the potential of its IC.

The fetus, moreover, is recognized by the mother's body as foreign enough for her immune system to start up its self-protective chemicals. Promptly, though, her body suppresses half of these chemicals, lest she totally reject the fetus and thus miscarry.‡

A random biological mismatch, therefore, may be the cause of otherwise inexplicable miscarriages. People used to say, "It's a wise child that knows its own father." Today they might say, "It's a wise fetus that knows how to get along with its own mother." As Dr. Justin D. Call, chief of pediatric psychiatry at the University of California at Irvine, says, "We no longer think of the newborn as a blank slate: the infant is already the veteran of an intimate set of interactions between itself, the mother, and the placenta, which affect both physiology and psychology."

Differences between twins start early in uterine life. Each twin, for example, attaches itself to a different section of the placenta, thus receiving a different amount of blood supply. As a result, twins are almost

*Willard Gaylin, *Caring* (New York: Avon, 1979).
†James A. Joseph, "Black Americans in Africa," printed by the African American Institute, New York City, February 18, 1976.
‡When fetal cells are removed from the placental area where they have been wholesomely interracting with one half of the mother's immune system and are put into a laboratory dish with the second half which she has been suppressing, the combination of the two kills the fetal cells.

never the same weight at birth. Sometimes, in fact, one will be born normal while the other is but a tiny wizened corpse. When twins are both well and energetic, they spend months jockeying for position within the womb, with one of them necessarily emerging first. And after birth, they are likely to be treated somewhat differently by their parents. Unconsciously, the parents tend to respond with attraction or repulsion to the surprising power of each infant's IC, or the parent who sees one twin being favored by the other parent may unconsciously compensate by favoring the second twin.

Immediately after birth, the mammalian bonding process between infant and parent(s) begins. Today, skin contact is believed to be an important early part of that bonding. The newborn, even before the cord is cut, may be laid on the mother's bare abdomen or given her breast. Fathers, too, are encouraged to hold the infant at the earliest opportunity. On the other hand, a recent study suggests that the father does better to nurture the new mother, thus helping her to bond well with the baby, rather than step up too fast and try to nurture the baby himself. He needs to take his cue from the mother lest any precipitant action by him arouse her antagonism, not only toward him, but also, perhaps, toward the baby.

On the other hand, babies who, because of prematurity or illness, cannot benefit from early physical contact with parent(s), usually manage to make up for it later on.

There is no question, however, that infants must be mothered by someone, whether female or male, adult or older child, in order for infantile brain cells to develop at their normal, very rapid pace. In the laboratory, rodents deprived of mothering end up with fewer brain cells, fewer connections between cells, and different proportions of neurochemicals than their normally treated colleagues.

Human infants need touch and talk, not just food. Indeed, talk may serve as symbolic and surrogate touch, as the common language suggests: "Let's stay in touch"; "I was touched to hear from her"; "It was a touching speech."

Being physically touched by one's fellows is essential to all primates. In a famous experiment in the late 1950s, Harry and Margaret Harlow, psychologists at the University of Wisconsin, took infant monkeys from their mothers a few hours after birth and kept them in a germ-free environment away from other monkeys. They were fed by remote control. After a year, when the monkeys were returned to the group, they were real losers. They neither played with the others nor indulged much in mutual grooming. When attacked, they did not defend themselves. On reaching sexual maturity, they did not mate—and the females who were artificially inseminated ignored their firstborn young.* By the time their fourth infant was born, however, their behavior became relatively normal.

Next, the Harlows gave a "terry-cloth mother" to each isolated baby monkey. This towel-covered wooden dummy could hold a nursing bottle. The baby developed a normal clinging response, but not much else. He needed contact with a socially active peer, at least for a few hours a day, for normal development.

Moreover, as Harry Harlow, together with Stephen J. Suomi, M.D., later discovered, many of the socially retarded monkeys could be returned to normality if, for six months, they were daily exposed to an aggressive monkey who was bent on interacting with them. According to Columbia University neurobiologist Eric R. Kandel, "The characteristics of a successful monkey 'therapist' may include an obstinate and truculent pursuit . . . until the . . . socially withdrawn monkey . . . responds . . . with an apparent flight into health—almost, as it were out of desperation."†

Among humans, early social deprivation can also often be compensated for, but there is no stage of life at which prolonged lack of contact with other human beings is not likely to weaken good health and spirits. Solitary confinement is one of the most dreaded of punishments. And many people are convinced that the large modern hospital, with its chilly, depersonalized setting, serves to delay healing.

One example is the intensive-care unit, where, for monitoring and treatment purposes, a severely ill patient may remain wired up to machines for days, weeks, even months. So sterile and mechanical is the atmosphere, so frightening the beepings and tickings that signal potential crisis that sometimes an emotional wounding (trauma) results that takes a further toll on the patient's health. In addition, the patient's family members may be emotionally injured by not having been prepared for the shock of seeing tubes gong into and wires sprouting out of their unspeaking, waxen loved one. This shock may take yet a further toll when it ricochets back onto the patient. Fears, like colds, are only too easily passed along, especially when the recipient is already in a weakened condition.

Hopelessness and hidden anger within one person may also resonate with—and reinforce—similar vibrations in another person, while the happier, more positive feelings are unconsciously tuned out. Here the term *vibration* is particularly apt. Not only do living creatures emanate

*Harry and Margaret Harlow, "The Nature of Love," *The American Psychologist*, Vol. 13, 1958.
†Eric R. Kandel, "Psychotherapy and the Single Synapse," *New England Journal of Medicine*, 8 November 1979.

measurable amounts of electromagnetic energy, but even inanimate objects tend to vibrate in unison when their rhythms approach similarity, a phenomenon called *entrainment*. As writer and editor George Leonard points out in *The Silent Pulse*, some young women who share an apartment start having their periods at the same time, and some clocks in a clock store start chiming simultaneously.

The unconscious meshing of two people's vibrations can be either negative or positive. "He brings out the best (or the worst) in me." Such synergism is reflected in other ordinary phrases: "We're on the same wavelength"; "The chemistry was right"; "We see things in the same light."

When mutually reinforcing love between two people continues, it may so expand and intertwine their boundaries that they "feel as one"; indeed, sometimes they grow to look alike. Karl Menninger, the renowned psychiatrist, when speaking of his wife of more than fifty years, said, "We're not just married; we're fused."

On the other hand, children sometimes grow up with parents who feel little affinity with them. (This appears to have been the case with Dorothy.) The parents may be athletes and the child an intellectual, or vice versa; the parents may have one kind of humor and the child another. Sometimes mutual understanding arises out of their differences, but at other times the child may feel closer to a grandparent than to the parents, or the parents may have to wait for their own grandchild before feeling they have a soulmate in the family. Some parents force themselves to voice more affection for a child than they genuinely feel. On the other hand, some children are so hungry for adult affection that they see evidence of it even in behavior not thus intended. Pitiful, for example, is the way some abused children keep on blaming themselves, rather than their parent(s), for the parental violence against them. They insist that somehow they must have deserved the brutal punishment. It is as if they wished to keep intact the imaginary archetype of the loving parent, even at the expense of their own self-image—or their physical safety.

No human parents, no matter how devoted, can love all their children equally all the time. The best that any child with siblings can hope for is that the parents have different favorites at different times of the day or year, with each child eventually given approximately equal time in the sun.

Though much has been written about the damage to the child who feels parental rejection, more is being discovered about the kind of damage suffered by the parental favorite. Sometimes the favorite grows up with unconscious terror of jealousy on the part of the other parent, not to mention siblings; sometimes the favorite, like a self-appointed Atlas, is unconsciously convinced that upon his shoulders rests the responsibility for the parents' happiness or the preservation of the marriage.

It was Dr. Alfred Adler, one of psychiatry's founding fathers and himself the youngest of four sons, who suggested the importance of sibling rivalry in mental health. (Not surprisingly, Freud, an eldest child, focused more on the child's relationship with parents.) Long after the siblings have grown up, their rivalry may continue unabated, at least at an unconscious level.

Just as children tend to see their parents through the veil of archetype, so do parents tend to see their child through a veil of ambition, symbolic or real, for themselves or the family. In the U.S., expectations are higher than elsewhere for children to surpass their parents. Because of chronic unemployment, this goal is more difficult to achieve than formerly. As a result, many young adults suffer from profound frustration. Some go as far as to express their disappointment in the polluted status quo by engaging in behavior that is destructive to themselves or others.

It is a rarity for parents to be consistently compatible with offspring throughout their growth. When parent and child find themselves at loggerheads, time may be their ally. Nor is there need for parents to bring their child fully into their confidence when the vibrations between them feel jarring. "Let it all hang out" is dubious advice at best, even between consenting adults, and may be seriously counterproductive when riled parents are too explicit with a child about the dismay he is causing them.

As for receiving unspoken messages, there is evidence that accuracy of this type of perception is greater among females than males. It is also greater among parents than childless couples.* Some infants, however, seem to have been born without the capacity to receive or give appropriate emotional feedback. No matter how much devotion a parent genuinely lavishes on them, they do not respond.

These children have been termed *mother-killers*, and some pediatricians believe that a recessive gene or subclinical brain malformation or damage may underlie the baby's tragic inability to metabolize love.

Some children who are truly deprived of love stretch and bend, like plants toward the sun, and somehow manage to get the love they need at some stage from some person. Other children who do not receive the specific signs of love they want from a particular individual may wilt. Yet unlike childhood rickets, which permanently injures the bone deprived of calcium, childhood deprivation of a particular kind of love is

*J. A. Hall, R. Rosenthal, D. Archer, M. R. DiMatteo, P. L. Rogers, "Decoding Wordless Messages," *Human Nature*, May 1978.

often made up for later. What Chicago psychoanalyst Franz Alexander named "the corrective emotional experience" may occur through friendship or courtship, a fortunate confluence of needs with another person, or through therapy. For example, a valued person's warm acceptance of oneself *as one is* may interrupt and reverse an old vicious cycle of feeling unloved and consequently driven to behave in unlovable or unloving ways (as Dorothy continued to do). Even the terry-cloth-raised monkey females became affectionate by the time their fourth baby came along.

Another kind of corrective emotional experience may result when an individual is assured that his parents, who have been unrelentingly critical of him, should themselves be criticized for being overly perfectionist (as was the case with Sanford's father). Because the impact of impossible parental expectation is thus diluted, the individual may reduce his agonizing self-hate based on necessarily failing to fulfill this expectation.

Several men who managed to make up in later life for emotionally wounding childhoods were described by Dr. George Vaillant in *Adaptation to Life*, his book about a long-term study of 141 Harvard graduates from the early 1940s. Some of the happiest and healthiest men had suffered as children under alcoholic, even abusive, parents. The urge to compensate for what they had missed led them to behave in a loving, sensitive way toward their own wives and offspring and also to achieve success at work.* But other men with similarly unfortunate childhoods continued to suffer throughout adulthood. In time their inability to get along with people became exacerbated by serious psychosomatic symptoms, and vice versa, in a vicious cycle, so that many died earlier than their classmates. Dr. Vaillant comments, "What makes or breaks our 'luck' seems to be the continued interaction between our choice of adaptive mechanisms and our sustained relationships with other people."

In family relationships, Vaillant says, there is one thing even worse for children than parental rejection, alcoholism, child abuse, or desertion (whether through death, or physical or psychological distancing). This is a parent who is so thoroughly unpredictable that the child is kept perpetually off-balance, able neither to remain safely attached nor cleanly to break free. As Vaillant says, "No whim of fate, no Freudian trauma, no loss of a loved one, will be as devastating to the human spirit [IC] as some prolonged ambivalent relationship that leaves us forever unable to say goodbye." Dr. Fred Plum, chief of neurology at New York Hospital, sees similar danger from "the parent who keeps promising rewards and producing punishments."

---

*According to Freud, the two criteria for mental health are in fact the abilities to work and love (*arbeiten und lieben*).

Some ambivalence is natural, of course, to a creature subject to the perpetual motion of his own and other people's four dimensions and "three brains." A parent whose child has just taken an unnecessary risk may want simultaneously to hug and hit it. But prolonged extreme parental ambivalence may tear the child apart by forcing him into what anthropologist Gregory Bateson called the *double-bind*.

Then trouble comes no matter which choice the person makes—or even if he makes no choice at all. An example is the old ditty: " 'Mother, may I go in for a swim?'/ 'Yes, my darling daughter./ Hang your clothes on a hickory limb,/ but don't go near the water.' "

In a double-bind, the person feels both immobilized and diminished; whatever he does—or does not do—is likely to produce guilt. One way to escape a bind, at least temporarily, is through the unconscious defense of humor. Both immobilized individuals and captive populations have mobilized their respective IC's sufficiently well to gain through "gallows humor" a refreshing perspective on a tragic situation that they are powerless to change. Another way is to force oneself to cease caring so avidly any longer about the subject of the bind or the binding person himself. There are times when a cultivated indifference (one form of distancing) can be "just what the doctor ordered."

It is also well to guard against unwittingly placing others in a double-bind (one theory is that the individual who keeps putting others in a bind may feel himself in one). On the other hand, some professionals deliberately use the bind in a therapeutic manner. Psychologist Paul Watzlawick tells of a patient who found it impossible to say no to people. He asked her to stand up in front of her group. "Say no," he commanded.

If she refused or was silent, she was, in effect, saying no to him. If she obeyed, she was gaining practice in saying no.*

Different from the double-bind is alternating between one state of mind and another. Not only is this a normal procedure for humans, but it also conforms to the basic rhythm of nature. Within the body, for example, the heartbeat is divided into systole and diastole; within the mind, there are waking and sleeping; within the environments, there are night and day, stillness and motion, rain and shine, and the many factors characterized as yin and yang. Within human relationships, there are:
• talking and listening
• seeking company and solitude
• playing front-stage and working behind the scenes
• being dependent and independent
• committing oneself and hanging loose

*Paul Watzlawick, *The Language of Change*, New York, Basic Books, 1978.

- distancing oneself and moving closer
- being firm and pliant
- fighting and giving in

Within a relationship, whether of a couple or family or other small group, *feedback from people* provides for the individual's social dimension what homeostasis does for the body, and what unconscious defenses do for the mind. Personal comments that are unambiguously offered and accurately received provide a gyroscope for the ship of relations (or relation*ship*).

"The best mirror," as the poet George Herbert said, "is a good friend." And the care and feeding of one's close relationships is a major health measure. Even the care and feeding of a pet has been found to increase longevity, both through the responsibility assumed by the person and the drop in his blood pressure that has been observed to occur when humans address a loved animal.

In a wholesome human relationship, the partners unconsciously keep balancing each other. If one is feeling dependent, the other may take charge; if one is being taciturn, the other may speak up; if one is weary, the other may exhibit a surge of energy.*

In couples who remain happy, according to Yale psychologist Robert Sternberg, there is relative parity in the degree of their love for one another. This parity may be among the factors that enable the pair to keep pinch-hitting for one another.

By the 1940s, psychiatrist Harry Stack Sullivan had moved beyond Freud's emphasis on the importance for the patient's mental health of the key adults in his past. Instead, Sullivan stressed the importance of people *here and now*, both as individuals and as comembers of the patient's small group, such as family (family is defined by anthropologist Ashley Montague as "a place for shared genes to keep warm in a cold world"). At about the same time, the importance of the broader society of which the family itself is part was stressed by such psychological experts as Wilhelm Reich, Erich Fromm, Karen Horney, and Melanie Klein.

Today, family therapy is the fastest-growing branch of professional help in the United States. Because a family comprises a system, a change in one part may affect the whole; indeed, even a change in the *relationship* of one part to another part may change the whole. Therapists sometimes ask to see not only the patient's parents or siblings, mate or child, but also grandparents—even the family pet. The hypothesis is that the pa-

---

*In rare instances, however, two people, rather than balancing each other, reinforce each other's offbeat fantasies to such a degree that the two as a unit go out of sync with the rest of the world (*folie à deux*). Such couples fail to provide healthful feedback to each other and also join in rejecting healthful feedback from the outside.

thology is less *within* one family member than *between* family members.

Just as the body may have a target organ, so a family may have a target person—one whose behavior symbolizes the emotional difficulties of the others. Sometimes he (or she) serves as a scapegoat, thus perhaps freeing other siblings from parental wrath; sometimes he is forced to be quiet because the others refuse to pay attention to what he has to say; sometimes his dependence is useful for those family members whose self-esteem derives almost entirely from their need to be needed.

Whatever the family pattern, it is likely to be clung to: "This is the way we Smiths have always done things." Yet some change in the family as a unit may be necessary lest the reaction by parents or siblings to improvement in the health (or behavior) of the target person be an unfortunate one. A too-possessive parent, for example, may respond to new independence in the patient by developing symptoms of his own.

Family therapy, like other group endeavors, is not for every patient. When someone's inner balance is too precarious, or when the unconscious defenses are used in too paranoid a manner ("You only say that because you hate me"), then even the most accurate feedback may be useless—or worse ("You've always hated me, so I'll do the opposite of what you want"). For some people (like Dorothy) an inner change feels so threatening that whoever suggests it must be wishing her ill.

JUNE: Did Dorothy's father rally 'round after her husband was killed?

NORMAN: Not enough. Peter made an extra effort, but their relationship had not evolved with the years. To him she was still a small child who needed to be set straight, rather than a grieving woman who needed emotional support.

JUNE: And her psychiatrist?

NORMAN: The psychiatrist had a hard time with her own dislike of Dorothy.

JUNE: What did she do?

NORMAN: She worked on herself. In fact, she asked a colleague to give her some professional sessions. One possibility was to refer Dorothy to another psychiatrist. But finally Dorothy's doctor learned to feel better about Dorothy. She then suggested that Dorothy join the therapy group she was codirecting.

JUNE: Codirecting?

NORMAN: Yes. Groups are often most effective when led by male and female cotherapists.

JUNE: What was Dorothy's response?

NORMAN: She accused the doctor of trying to worm more money out of her.

JUNE: What could the doctor do?

NORMAN: She was in a bind. If she didn't try to get Dorothy into group, she'd be backing down from what she considered optimal treatment. But when she did try, Dorothy accused her of financial greed.

JUNE: How did the psychiatrist handle it?

NORMAN: As people *can* handle a bind: first by identifying it as such, then by setting a fair limit to their own efforts. For her, this meant facing the fact that no doctor can help a patient who is determined to stay sick and refuses to accept responsibility for any of her predicaments.

JUNE: What can you do when people get furious at the slightest suggestion that some change in themselves may be needed?

NORMAN: Try the "I message." Say, "*I* am confused when you do this," not "*You* are a jerk for doing this." That way, you don't get their hackles up so much, or their defenses. They may actually hear you. Another thing is to try to stimulate the person's capacity for joy: Find something he would like, and then tie the suggestion for change to that something. The ability to feel pleasure provides an important inner motive toward health. For example, if Dorothy had enjoyed active sports, then losing weight in order to jog better might have inspired her to diet. But, unfortunately, she didn't care at all about sports, or much about people. Trying to earn someone else's approval may provide a major motive to change one's ways.

JUNE: But didn't Dorothy value her husband's approval?

NORMAN: Yes. For a time; within limits. George admired her hair and skin, and he appreciated the financial security she provided.

JUNE: Yet he refused when she begged him to visit her doctor.

NORMAN: Perhaps he was afraid. Perhaps he didn't want to discuss why he had married a woman who was letting herself grow more unattractive every year.

JUNE: Why do you suppose he did marry her?

NORMAN: Hard to tell. At some level, he might have figured that no one was likely to compete with him, so his sexual performance wouldn't have to be all that great.

JUNE: Do many men reason like that?

NORMAN: Today, particularly, when there's so much emphasis on performance as the goal.

JUNE: Why did Dorothy go into such a panic when she started feeling better and losing weight? I should think that would have been the beginning of a wholesome cycle.

NORMAN: It might have been. But unconsciously she had become so reliant on her symptom that its change threw her emotional economy off-kilter. You often see this kind of temporary anxiety when big changes occur in any dimension. After all, it also hurts to have a broken bone set correctly, but the short-term pain is worth the long-term healing.

JUNE: Especially in regard to our relationships with people?

NORMAN: They are worth a big investment of effort and time. Our human environment, like the ecological kind, is more important to our well-being than many people used to think.

VI
Mostly Relationships With Environments
Introducing Peter

*"Changes in the social structures and personal be-
havior patterns . . . will do far more than doctors
and drugs can to minimize the burden of disease. . . . Better health may require, for instance,
land reforms in El Salvador, the control of air pollution in Japan, and well-digging programs in rural
India; dietary changes in the United States, a cut
in cigarette smoking in Scotland, and the control
of cotton dust in an Egyptian textile factory."*
—*Erik P. Eckholm*, The Picture of Health

Peter, Dorothy's father, is seventy. The southern textile factory for
which he worked from age fifteen to sixty-five supplements his social
security with a meager pension. Once he sued the company for
disability benefits because of suspected brown-lung disease. But the
doctors, though admitting that Peter had a serious cough, attributed
it to his smoking in the present, rather than to inhaling cotton dust
in the past. They told him to give up his several packs a day.

"They can't ruin my pleasures," he told his friend Anthony. "It's
bad enough having them ruin my health."

Actually, Peter could not remember ever feeling really well. His
mother had died when he was two, and he had grown up in a share-
cropper household where food was inadequate. He never grew as
tall as his two older brothers, who were born before the family income
diminished; and by the time he was thirty, Peter's teeth were gone.
Still, he retained a wiry strength and is pleased to have reached a
greater age than his two brothers or his father ever did.

Peter's apartment faced on an alley. The rent was low because of the daily noise from an automotive repair shop. Peter complained to his daughter Dorothy that he could not afford a better place because of the alimony he still had to pay to "that bitch," Martha.

One August morning his friend Anthony appeared as usual, and knocked. No answer. He knocked again. From inside he could hear some stirring. The door was unlocked, so he went in. There stood Peter, nude, unshaven, glassy-eyed, amid a shambles of broken crockery and furniture. His knuckles and toes were bleeding from all his punching and kicking. "They're choking me," he shouted—and then crumpled to the floor.

Anthony phoned for an ambulance and pulled a pair of pants onto Peter.

At the hospital, the diagnosis was senile psychosis with paranoid mentation. Also, Peter's blood pressure was far too high. He was given a tranquilizer and a diuretic. He complained of dizziness and a ringing in his ears. Gradually, his drug dosage was reduced, and by midwinter he seemed fine. It was a happy day when Dorothy came to escort him home. And he remained well for half a year.

Over the week of July fourth, Anthony was out of town.

By the time he returned and went to visit Peter, he found him on the floor, whimpering. "My head hurts," Peter said. He had been vomiting.

Again Anthony brought him to the hospital. Again Peter's health gradually improved. Again he was sent home.

One hot misty Indian-summer day, Dorothy found him coughing more than usual and looking pallid. Her first fear was of a stroke, because, as she knew, the symptoms of Transient Ischemic Attack (TIS) include hypertension, headache, and periods of disorientation. She marched over to the open window and shouted to the mechanic to take it easy with the hammering.

"Listen, lady," he shouted back, "this is my job."

She slammed the window.

"Don't do that," Peter said. "I'm stifling."

"You're right. I've got a headache myself."

"Those bastards never *would* install an exhaust fan," he said. "They never gave a shit about their workers." And he dropped to the floor.

Again he was taken to the hospital; again he improved. Then Martha, his former wife, died. Without the need to pay alimony, Peter could afford a nicer apartment. Unfortunately, its location meant a long trip for Anthony. But Peter's health remained stable.

*   *   *

Human beings, with their adaptive capacities and intelligence can live in the Arctic and the tropics, the rain forest and the desert, and in weird artificial environments such as those of space modules and deep-sea diving bells. Much of our adaptive capacity is unconscious and automatic: we quite literally don't give it a thought. One example is the way many Indians living high in the Andes develop extra-large lungs.

Among the factors that influence our adaptability is timing. Science writer Gay Gaer Luce, author of *Body-Time*, has concluded that "the rhythmic nature of earth life is, perhaps, its most usual yet overlooked property." The waxings and wanings to which we are subject include such forces as gravity, electromagnetism, radiation, light, and sound. The turning of the earth upon its axis provides night and day; its annual turning around the sun provides seasonal cold and warmth; its relationship to the moon provides thirteen twenty-eight-day cycles per year.*

Living creatures, from lizards to marigolds, share with humans a twenty-four-hour, or circadian (*circa dies* means "about a day"), rhythm of activity and rest. This rhythm affects every system of the body, probably every cell. Sometimes all our rhythms are in sync with each other and those of the outside world, and we feel wonderful. Other times these rhythms are in conflict. "This is not my day," we may apologize.

For humans, being prevented from experiencing even a symbolic form of night and day is felt as cruel deprivation. As demoralizing as solitary confinement may be imprisonment in a room with unremitting bright light—or no light at all.

Within the twenty-four hours, there are predictable variations in human metabolism. People are likely to be at their most alert after breakfast. After lunch, however, their alertness is likely to drop. Yet individuals vary tremendously as to which part of the circadian cycle is best for their internal systems. "I'm a night person," one will say, or "I do my most creative work in the morning." A common example of one's systems being out of sync is jet lag. Not only may the person feel subjectively out of sorts, but objectively, too, there are changes in his normal fluctuations of blood pressure, pulse, temperature, and respiration; his bloodstream's sugar, hemoglobin, minerals, and hormones; his brain and nervous system's biochemicals; even the rate at which his cells divide.

Another example is a too-rapid change in work shifts. Though our body "clocks" do reset themselves, they need time to adjust to any new

---

*The length of each cycle is mirrored by human menstruation. More controversial is the claim by some cosmobiologists that the full moon (lune) coincides every twenty-eight days with a rise in human mental illness (lunacy) and violent crime.

routine. Jane Brody, health columnist of the *New York Times*, points to the haunting fact that the Three Mile Island catastrophe took place with a crew that had just rotated to the night shift and at an hour, 4:00 A.M., when most people are at their least alert and slowest to respond to a signal of warning. (4:00 A.M. is also the hour when most babies are born. Said *New Yorker* writer Ved Mehta, whose own daughter had chosen that time, "We may be nocturnal animals after all.")

Experiments done with laboratory animals reveal a surprising hazard in exposing them to too much stress at the time of day when they are naturally at their *most* alert. Summing up these findings, Gay Gaer Luce writes: "Life and death may hang in the balance of timing. Mortality has been decided, experimentally, not by the amount, but by the time of day that a rodent received x-rays or was injected with pneumonia virus, bacteria, or drugs. Exposure to loud noise affects a rodent little during his period of rest, but may hurtle him into a frenzy . . . and even death, if it occurs during his activity period."*

In humans, experiments at the University of Minnesota show that some cancer drugs have more beneficial impact, with fewer side effects, if given at a particular time of day.

Observation of humans also suggests that there is controllable rhythm in the highs and lows of some manic-depressive patients. They feel fine in summer but crippled by despondency in winter, when daylight is at its lowest intensity and duration. Such patients seem to benefit from exposure in winter to fluorescent bulbs (the kind of "growth light" used with plants). Says MIT's Richard J. Wurtman, M.D., "We are all unwitting subjects of a long-term experiment on the effects of artificial lighting on health; until much more is known, we should design indoor lighting to resemble as closely as possible what the sun provides."

Light, after all, has long been manipulated by farmers to increase egg and milk production. And more recently, with humans, light has been successfully used to treat jaundice in newborns and psoriasis in people of all ages. It is also being used experimentally to fight herpes and some forms of cancer. Hospital architects are even beginning to place windows in intensive-care units, while different wall colors are being used to bring out different moods. Some hospitals and prisons, for example, now have an all-pink room to calm violent patients, while some restaurant designers believe that dark red stimulates the appetite.

Too much sunlight, however, may be harmful to the skin (and to unprotected eyes). Though most skin cancers are so self-contained and

*Gay Gaer Luce, "Biological Rhythms in Psychiatry and Medicine," *National Institutes of Mental Health Bulletin*, 1970.

slow-growing that there is no rush about removing them, others, such as melanoma, should be promptly and deeply excised.*

Radiation is inescapably part of the human environment, sometimes doing good, sometimes harm. Everything, including the human body and brain, emits it. From outer space come gamma rays and X rays; from powerlines comes enough low-level radiation to cause laboratory mice to alter their behavior (by trying to escape it). Other radiation sources include microwave ovens, color televisions, and automatic garage doors.

A further factor with probable influence on human health is the way some gas molecules (air ions) take on an electrical charge when cosmic forces bombard the earth or when local forces—such as ocean waves, waterfalls, and bubbling springs—fling water droplets into the air. The long-term popularity of spas reflects the belief that there are health benefits in the charge thus given to the air-ions.

Sound waves, too, can affect health. A comparison between ten thousand people living near the Los Angeles airport and a control group farther away showed that among the nearby people aged seventy-five and over, the number of deaths from heart attack and stroke was 18 percent higher than in the control group, and that the suicide rate of people forty-five to fifty-five was double that of the control group.† An example of sound's benefits is the way newborns tend to eat and sleep better if the nursery clock ticks loudly at seventy-two beats a minute, the familiar rate of the maternal heart.

Because the individual's adaptation response to environmental stress is so often unconscious and automatic, it is likely to be unselective. It may therefore need some IC supervision or comment from other people to bring it into line with good health practice. Sometimes an under-adaptation needs to be increased; sometimes an overadaptation needs to be curbed. An Andean Indian whose lungs had not sufficiently expanded might need access to oxygen or training in maximal breathing; a worker who runs a jackhammer all day and turns the radio up when he gets home may need a family member to shout, "What's the matter with you? Are you *deaf*?" Peter, as soon as he could afford to, moved away from his old apartment, where his worst problems had occurred in summer, when, although his windows admitted air and light, they also admitted noise and polluted air from the garage.

Some forms of environmental stress derive not only from one's immediate neighborhood but also from one's geographical region. Many

*Patients may need to remind their doctor to view all skin surfaces at the time of a routine physical exam.
†Report by The Acoustical Society of America, May 10, 1983.

parts of the world are subject to annual long-lasting one-directional winds (*khamsin* in Israel, *mistral* in France, *Foehn* in Germany, *sirocco* in Italy, *meltamie* in Greece, and *Santa Ana* in California). So taken for granted is the malevolent effect of such a wind on human mood and behavior that in some of these countries, serious crimes, including rape and murder, draw lighter sentences if committed at that time of year. And local doctors prepare to be overworked especially in the poorer districts, where flimsy homes provide inadequate protection against the wind and clouds of dust accompanying it.

Although humans share their natural environment with the rest of the animal kingdom, they have also created a pervasive second environment—namely, civilization. And the health effects of the second rival, even sometimes exceed, those of the first. In the mid-nineteenth century, Karl Marx startled the world by pointing to people's economic class as central to their values and hence their behavior. In the mid-twentieth century, computer-aided analysis startled the world by pointing to people's economic class as central to their health.

American blacks, for example, who are generally poorer than whites, suffer more from such ailments as hypertension and cancer. They also tend to die many years earlier than whites of the same gender. Yet when blacks move into middle- or upper-class neighborhoods, their health profile becomes relatively indistinguishable from that of their white neighbors.

One remaining differential exemplifies how the same unselective, unconscious body reaction can be productive in one environment yet unproductive in another. Sickle-cell anemia, a hereditary disease among blacks, serves as protection against malaria. Had some of the African ancestors of today's American blacks not had that gene, they might not have survived long enough to reach this country. But now that this country is free of malaria, the sickle-cell anemia gene is a serious, even lethal, drawback, and many of today's prospective parents seek genetic counseling in order to avoid handing it down. Adoption is the path chosen by many of them.

Socially as well as economically, one's health is subject to influence by the culture into which one is born. As the Reverend Martin Luther King, Jr., said, "Creation is so designed that my personality can only be fulfilled in the context of community." Yet the wider American community spurned the racial group to which he belonged. The health hazards from this kind of negative feedback from the social environment were described by Dr. Eugene Brody, then president of the World Federation for Mental Health, in its 1982 bulletin: "A salient feature of being a member of a minority is that . . . discrimination, prejudice, and exclusion from opportunity are suffered because one happens to belong to a socially visible category of people. These inflicted wounds have in common the fact that they are dehumanizing. . . . This constitutes a denial of one's unique past history and the individuality shaped by it, and of the reflective self-awareness [IC] crucial to being human."

In a landmark U.S. Supreme Court decision in 1964, *Brown v. Board of Education*, existing schools for young "negroes" were judged to be *not* equal to those of whites, because they were separate. Taken into account by the justices was evidence from the social and psychological sciences that to be discriminated against, particularly during one's formative years, can itself be an impediment to healthy development. Just as a dread form of individual punishment is solitary confinement, so, for a group, is being legally ostracized, as is still the case for the blacks in South Africa.

In the U.S., unfortunately, custom has not kept up with the growing number of laws for social and economic justice. Unemployment for blacks is far greater than for whites, especially for young males, half of whom, in some areas, cannot find jobs. Residential areas for blacks are often worse than those for whites in terms of air and noise pollution and frequency of crime. Though blacks in increasing numbers have left such backgrounds behind, the average American black is still at a disadvantage, compared to the average white, in terms of health.

While the 1960s saw American discriminatory laws against blacks stricken from the books, the 1970s saw the same new justice applied to women. As women's job opportunities have increased, so, it appears, has their well-being. Says Grace Baruch, a psychologist at Wellesley College, "Equality . . . leads . . . to mental health."

This improvement applies particularly to those women whose jobs are good enough to give them an IC sense of mastery. Many such women in their middle years have been studied by psychiatrist Jean Baker Miller, author of *Toward a New Psychology of Women*. Theirs, she says, is "a new sense of self and a new burst of energy." Nor are they as depressed as middle-aged women traditionally have been by the sense of "fading attractiveness" and "the feeling that their lives are over."

Dr. Miller attributes this new vigor to the women's movement although, as she says, "The issues that feminism raises are so deep and so ancient that we would be thinking simplistically to expect things to change quickly." Furthermore, only relatively few women (and men) attain top jobs, which leaves most women working for low pay and little chance of advancement.

The discombobulation felt by men because of women's recent rise in status may be one reason that 10 percent more American men are turning to psychotherapy in the 1980s than the 1970s.* Yet some men report feeling the better for their new freedom from needing to be the family's sole breadwinner; they also enjoy society's new "permission" to express their so-called feminine and nurturing side. But other men report feeling upset, threatened, and depressed. This is painful not only for them but also, ironically, for the women in their lives.

The overfeminization of young children is a new kind of environmental hazard. The Secretary of Health of Puerto Rico was so alarmed by reports of premature sexual development in thousands of small girls that on January 17, 1985, he appointed an expert panel to pinpoint the cause(s). Under suspicion are estrogen and other substances fed to cattle and poultry to fatten them. Some infant girls have developed breasts, pubic hair, and have begun to menstruate; a few infant boys have developed breasts. In 40 percent of the cases, the symptoms disappear if the child is no longer fed milk, eggs, or other edibles containing chemical growth stimulants. Ironically, the hormone that stimulates growth in animals and poultry ultimately stunts human growth because bone development slows after puberty, no matter how early puberty begins. About 50 percent of the meat consumed in Puerto Rico comes from Central America, where laws against selling animal products saturated with growth chemicals are not enforced as they are on the American mainland and theoretically within Puerto Rico itself.

An individual's health is subject not only to conflicts of interest within his society but also to conflicts between his society and others. If, for example, people must fight for their country in a good cause—as happened, most agree, with the Allies in World War II—then, if they are not killed or badly wounded, they may feel better than they ever have, or ever will again, for it is one of life's major invigorations to know that one is an integral part of something more significant than oneself. If, however, the war is viewed by many people as unjustifiable, as the Vietnam War came to be, then someone who fought in it may deeply suffer, in mind or body, in relationships with people and with the home environment. (By 1985 the death rate, as well as illness rate, of Vietnam veterans was considerably higher than for other veterans and the rest of the population.)

Although hypocrisy has been called "the tribute that vice pays to virtue," and a bit of it certainly greases the wheels of social exchange, it may also corrode the well-being of those people who are continually

---

*And counselors at colleges and universities have reported a notable increase in the number of male students seeking help against impotence.

forced to make use of it. This is particularly true when the kind of individual liberty necessary for IC development is also restricted. As Boris Pasternak has Yurii say in *Doctor Zhivago*, "Your health is bound to be affected if, day after day, you say the opposite of what you feel, if you grovel before what you dislike. . . . Our nervous system isn't just a fiction, it's part of our physical body, and it can't be forever violated with impunity."

On the other hand, as some flower children and their successors in the "me generation" discovered, too few restrictions may also lead to individual health damage, whether in body or mind, as often happened through unbridled use of drugs, or in human relationships, as often happened through unbridled narcissism. One possible explanation for the way license promotes damage to health is offered by philosophy professor Andrew Oldenquist of Ohio State University: "We are born ready and receptive to be limited and molded by rules, ethics, ritual, manners and tradition, and we go bad when our society—our tribe— neglects to limit and mold us in these ways. We go bad because this is a form of rejection. We are rejected as surely when we are not held accountable . . . as when we are denied food or shelter."*

Oldenquist therefore proposes a year of compulsory national service for everyone at age eighteen. Though pay would be low, the experience would assure young women as well as men "that they belonged and were needed."

There is no doubt that some social improvement for youth is needed in this country, where the rate for automobile and other accidents among youths aged fifteen to twenty-five is rising, and suicide has become the third leading cause of death in that age group, as well as eighth among even younger children (five to fourteen). Seatbelt and motorcycle-helmet laws are public-health measures in the right direction, but much remains to be done by individuals, families, and society.

Alarming, too, is the way substance abuse, whether nicotine or alcohol, psychedelic or hard drugs, has risen in recent years while the age of its onset has dropped. True, there are major frustrations in the lives of many contemporary young people, such as unemployment and a dearth of what Oldenquist characterizes as tribally-assigned responsibility. These, furthermore, are overarched by the nuclear threat, which arouses doubt in many young people as to whether they will even *have* a future. Says Tim Page, a successful young music writer, "The members of my age group came to maturity believing—silently but profoundly—that these were the final days; that we were to have no sequel. Our fear of immediate

Newsweek, "My Turn," 5 April 1982.

extinction has caused many of us to pass through life as though it were an endless Sunday brunch, grasping out halfheartedly at trends and textures. I have spent my share of time mouthing the platitudes of nihilism, while secretly frightened of caring too deeply. If you hold on to nothing, little can be taken from you."*

When Yale psychiatrist Robert J. Lifton interviewed large numbers of college students, he found that their dreams were riddled with imagery reflecting a terror of the nuclear holocaust. Though some individuals had not been aware of harboring this terror, nonetheless it infiltrated their other attitudes, including perhaps that of recklessness toward their own current or future health.

Paradoxically, a similar recklessness among young people may be engendered by the very monotony of their lifelong good health. These, after all, are the first people in history to get through childhood without the high fevers and other IC-jolting threats to life that formerly were commonplace and, in some instances, served to stimulate spiritual growth. It may, therefore, not be entirely coincidence that the first generation to grow up with the antimicrobial drugs should also be the first to turn on with psychedelics.

The most pitiful form of early onset of drug addiction is that of babies born to heroin-addicted mothers. For six weeks the infants need to go through all the pain of drug withdrawal.

In a partial sense, the first environment for everyone is another person (i.e., his mother.) And any extreme or prolonged stresses she is subjected to may have impact on the fetus. Experiments show that pregnant rats exposed to continuous severe overcrowding are more likely than others to produce offspring both with physical disabilities, such as cleft palate, and psychological ones, such as extreme timidity. Furthermore, male rats born to a mother subjected to extreme stress during her final stages of pregnancy often fail to develop the expected response to adult females when they reach maturity. Some scientists wonder if, similarly, some people's homosexuality may be related to their mothers' having been unduly stressed during late pregnancy. In all events, a useful development in science is the pinpointing of the time during pregnancy when various characteristics have their genesis. Thus, specific defects may sometimes be prevented if the mother-to-be takes special care during the corresponding stages.

Following birth, the mother still, to a considerable extent, mediates the child's environment, especially if she is nursing. According to

*Tim Page, "Life Miscarried," *The New York Times Magazine*, 27 January 1985.

Dr. W. Allen Walker of Harvard Medical School, when the mother nuzzles the baby, she breathes in and swallows his germs. Antibodies to them are then made in the lining of her intestinal tract. Directed by her hormones, these antibodies travel breastward, and the baby imbibes them with the milk. Inside the baby, the antibodies proceed to attack bacteria, viruses, and other substances that might otherwise cause infection or allergy. Statistically, breast-fed babies have fewer such problems than their bottle-fed contemporaries. Most of the latter, however, also thrive when lucky enough to be born in a land with easily obtainable refrigeration and parental literacy sufficient to understand the directions on an infant-formula package.

A new environmental hazard to children up to the age of nineteen is Reyes' syndrome, named for its Australian discoverer in 1963. It attacks young people just as they are recovering from certain other diseases, notably Type-B flu, chicken pox, a bad cold, or an intestinal bug (gastroenteritis). The onset of Reyes' syndrome, according to Georgetown University pediatrician Angel R. Colon, may be "like a tornado in the body. It wreaks havoc. It starts in the liver, affects the kidneys, the heart, the pancreas, the body muscles, and then creates brain swelling." The child must be rushed to a hospital. So dramatic are the symptoms, including relentless vomiting and unusual combativeness, that Dr. Colon finds it hard to believe that the great French and German pathologists of the nineteenth century would have missed this disease. His hypothesis for its arising today is that a formerly dormant virus has been activated by one or more of the pollutants resulting from industrial development. Thus may humankind indirectly suffer from its successes as well as its failures.*

As the 1984 Union Carbide tragedy in Bhopal, India, showed, some environmental pollutants can be immediately fatal. Others, like many carcinogens, take decades to show harmful effects. Yet clear health warnings about the latter continue to be ignored by people with the means to make a change in their environment or their habits. One reason is probably a natural inertia, but another may be the mixed messages received from the authorities. For example, the same U.S. government that insists on printing a warning on cigarette advertisements, that "smoking is dangerous to your health," also pays millions of dollars in subsidies to farmers to grow tobacco. And the latter continues despite the 1984 report by the Environmental Protection Agency naming "secondary" or "passive" to-

---

*Parents are cautioned against giving aspirin for the first disease, since there appears to be some connection between aspirin and the subsequent onset of Reyes' syndrome.

bacco smoke "the country's most dangerous airborne carcinogen," because of the statistics that show widows of smokers dying considerably earlier than widows of nonsmokers.

Tragic also is the continued gross injustice of health distribution, worldwide as well as at home. Whereas the United States can devote much of its medical research and treatment to the ailments of middle and old age—such as heart attack, stroke, and cancer—the less-developed countries cannot so much as handle the relatively easy-to-prevent child-killers, such as dysentery, cholera, and typhoid. Together, the latter are responsible for 80 percent of illness worldwide and for killing twenty million people a year. Nor can poor countries deal effectively with such lifelong disablers as malaria and other parasites. Within the United States, poor people, with fewer years of education than the affluent, are less well informed about preventive health measures, yet, with further injustice, they are also subject to worse environmental pollutants both at home and at work.

In the attempt to achieve a higher degree of health justice for Americans, during the last half of the 1970s the government tripled the number of health clinics for the poor. Ominous, however, have been the cutbacks in the 1980s of both clinics and childhood immunization programs against tetanus, diphtheria, polio, measles, and whooping cough. Warns Dr. Frederick C. Robbins, president of the Institute of Medicine at the National Academy of Sciences, "Most of the disease agents are still present in the population, just waiting for the number of susceptible children to become large enough that a wave of disease can sweep through them."*

Eternal vigilance, it seems, is the price not only of liberty but also of good health, for both oneself and one's descendants.

JUNE: What happened to Peter?

NORMAN: Well, you remember that his symptoms only appeared in summer when his windows were open?

JUNE: Was that the exhaust from cars?

NORMAN: In a way. But Peter's worst problem wasn't his lungs; it was his brain.

JUNE: His brain?

NORMAN: The kind of brain damage that is caused by an odorless, colorless gas—carbon monoxide.

*From a hearing of the House of Representatives' Energy and Commerce subcommittee on health, February 4, 1982.

JUNE: I thought that *killed* people.

NORMAN: It does if the quantity is large enough; otherwise it may give you a headache or ringing in the ears. You may vomit or become violent, the way Peter did.

JUNE: Does that happen often?

NORMAN: No, but probably more than people recognize. Everyone should beware of warming up a car in a closed garage, and should make sure their home heating vents are in good order.

JUNE: Yet Peter went right on living in that apartment even after he'd been hospitalized.

NORMAN: That's one of the toughest things about environmental illness. It's slow to develop, hard to recognize, and may aggravate the patient's problems in other dimensions, especially if he's elderly.

JUNE: How so?

NORMAN: It can make a symptom worse, like Peter's coughing. Or it can confuse the mind. Or it can add momentum to an unfortunate interpersonal cycle. The cough medicine Peter likes best is expensive; yet if he buys it, he won't have enough money to pay his ex-wife her full alimony; and the consequent rearousal of his old resentment against her makes his cough worse. Also his childhood had been a somewhat deprived one. It's during infancy and early childhood that the fundamentals of good health are laid down. Strong bones and teeth need calcium; emotional resilience needs consistent parenting. And Peter missed out. As for nutrition, rich people can afford both the protective foods and the junk food, but poor people are forced to choose, and often they choose wrong.

JUNE: I don't suppose TV helps, with ads that glamorize candies and colas, and ignore the wholesome foods.

NORMAN: Also, in poor families there's likely to be a parent missing, and the remaining parent must work very long hours. So the little kids are left to the mercies of an elder sibling or young aunt or uncle, and later may develop psychological problems that interfere with their earning power. People who grew up in poverty not only need to visit the doctor more often but miss more days of work. So the general vicious cycle of poverty leading to poor health leading to further poverty may march down through the generations.

JUNE: Was that true of Peter?

NORMAN: No. He was born feisty, with a potentially strong IC, and he worked hard to give his daughter, Dorothy, what he himself had never had: a good education. He was proud of that.

JUNE: But what about the diagnosis when he first went to the hospital: senile psychosis with paranoid mentation?

NORMAN: I hate that kind of label, and I use them as little as possible. The trouble is that insurance forms demand them. And it's true that in an emergency admission, the patient's listed category is of some help to the attending doctor.

JUNE: So Peter wasn't senile?

NORMAN: No. He was poisoned by that air.

JUNE: Was he paranoid?

NORMAN: Not as much as it seemed at first. Often there's an underlying structure to psychotic hallucination. Peter had been furious for years at his old bosses. Associating his current discomfort with his previous resentment at the conditions under which he had to work—*and* hold his tongue—he destroyed his own china and furniture.

JUNE: Is that kind of displaced violence common?

NORMAN: Not uncommon. And the urge toward violence is, at times, connected with the urge toward sex. The part of the brain where violence is mediated and the part for sex are very close together. This might explain why soldiers after battle so often commit rape. Or why TV so often includes violence and sex on the same program.

JUNE: But surely the IC has a role in both?

NORMAN: Always. And so does the conscience. That's why most people do *not* act out their forbidden sexual and violent wishes, except in dreams and fantasies. But the IC can be temporarily overwhelmed by stimuli from any or all the dimensions, as Peter's was when he went out of control. But then, if the IC is resilient, it brings the person back. The problem is that a strong IC is not always tied to virtue or good health. Some repeater criminals have a strong IC; they refuse to let anyone stop them from stealing back what they believe has been unfairly stolen from them. And some repeater patients are determined to enjoy their smoking and drinking to excess, no matter what anybody thinks. On the other hand, we also see virtuous hospital repeaters with, say, a fatal degenerative disease, who show such courage that every time members of the staff enter such a patient's room, they feel like saluting.

VII
The Intimate Connector

Introducing Jason

> "In view of the intimate connection between the things that we distinguish as physical and mental, we may look forward to a day when paths of knowledge . . . will be opened up, leading from organic biology and chemistry to the field of neurotic phenomena."
>
> —Freud, The Question of Lay Analysis
> (emphasis added)

Jason, a forty-year-old optometrist, found gray-eyed Mary Ellen the most attractive member of his therapy group. After he had teased her on the street about how angry she was, he invited her to lunch. After several months of dating, Jason began to feel better than he had since the death of his sister a year before.

At the time of his bereavement, he had moved from his apartment in his sister's old neighborhood, but he never managed to feel at home in the new place. He kept telling himself he would unpack his guitar music and the boxes of books, but he never got around to it. He signed up for an evening course in advanced optometry, and he kept making dates with new women. Despite jogging farther than usual, he had trouble sleeping. Feeling lethargic and apathetic, he lost interest in food, and when some of the women wanted to make love, he was occasionally impotent. He never played his guitar, and at work he had more and more trouble concentrating.

His internist ran him through a battery of tests. Strangely, Jason found himself dismayed when no serious abnormality showed up. A month later he insisted that the tests be rerun. This time, his liver function was abnormal enough for hepatitis to be suspected.

After two months of rest at home, his liver-function tests were normal, but he felt weaker than before. Was he suffering from the aftermath of hepatitis, or the debilitating effect of prolonged inactivity, or did he, as he was now convinced, have some rare disease involving the nervous system?

One night he awakened in a state of panic, his heart beating jerkily and fast. He phoned his best friend, Bill, a pharmacist. Bill came over, gave Jason a sleeping pill, and stayed with him the rest of the night.

Shortly thereafter, Bill and his wife, Nancy, dragooned Jason into coming along to their cottage at the beach.

However, Jason could not tolerate the sun. For the first time, it made him dizzy. He turned down Bill's invitations to go fishing, and he made no effort to get to know the young women Nancy invited over for drinks. (Because of the hepatitis, he drank no alcohol.) And he couldn't make sense out of the books he brought to study.

One night on the porch in the moonlight, Bill and Nancy, drinks in hand, administered to Jason the kind of verbal shock treatment that only a close friend or a trained therapist—or someone full of alcohol—is likely to attempt. They told him he was a pain in the neck, that he should knock off the self-pity, that he had become a drag on himself and everyone around him, and, in short, that he had better get himself into the hands of a psychiatrist.

Jason sat in icy silence. Then he rose. Psychiatry, he said, was full of crap—and so were they. With friends like them, he had no need of enemies. They should mind their own business.

Slowly, wearily, he headed down the beach. He did not return that whole night.

At dawn, Bill and Nancy set off to look for him. Nancy had been terrified that Jason would walk out into the ocean. Bill had insisted that Jason was safe; he was only punishing them.

It was Nancy who found him—sleeping in the lee of a dune. When she awakened him, he was somewhat confused. They walked back hand in hand. He told her that he had taken a long swim—far out beyond the reef, where none of them dared venture. It had seemed simplest not to turn back. But the full moon had come out from

behind a cloud. He felt that its beams were a kind of message—
directing him back to shore. The moment his feet touched sand, the
moon went under. What did she make of that?

Nancy was reminded of Hamlet's "There are more things in heaven
and earth, Horatio, than are dreamt of in your philosophy." But, she
said, before Jason fathomed all the deepest meanings of the universe,
they should pack, get home, and persuade Bill's psychiatrist friend,
Halston, to fit Jason into his crowded schedule.

The Intimate Connector is neither a substance nor an area; it is an
unconscious and conscious process that never ceases as long as a person
lives. During wakefulness and sleep, in kaleidoscopic fashion, the IC
organizes the four dimensions and their parts so as to form a pattern
characteristic of that individual. Spinoza might have been referring to
the IC when he said, "The effort by which each living thing endeavors
to persevere in its own being is nothing but the actual essence of the
thing itself."

"Its own being," for a human, includes awareness of himself as what
Arthur Koestler termed a *holon*. By this he meant the capacity of a whole
to be seen as a part, at the same time that any of its parts can be seen
as a whole. Take, for example, an organ or system of the body: In regard
to its specialized cells, it is a whole; yet in regard to its owner, it is a
part. Its owner, in turn, is a part, in regard to his family or nation; yet,
in regard to his four dimensions, his IC helps him feel and act as a
whole. Perhaps unique in the entire universe is the human individual
as a self-conscious unit who knows himself as sufficiently autonomous
to take responsibility for the health of his mind and body, yet dependent enough on other people and the environments that they can profoundly affect—for better or worse—the health of his mind and body
(see Fig. 3).

The IC can rise above itself (centrifugally) and also bring itself back
in touch with its own core (centripetally). Although these two directions
of functioning alternate, their degree of power is likely to remain constant. For it is when a person's IC is strong that he can extend himself
into far directions without impeding his return to the core of self.
But when his IC is weak, his outreach may be tentative and he may
—with accuracy—lack confidence in his power to return to the core of
self.

What a psychiatrist sometimes does is act as a temporary surrogate for

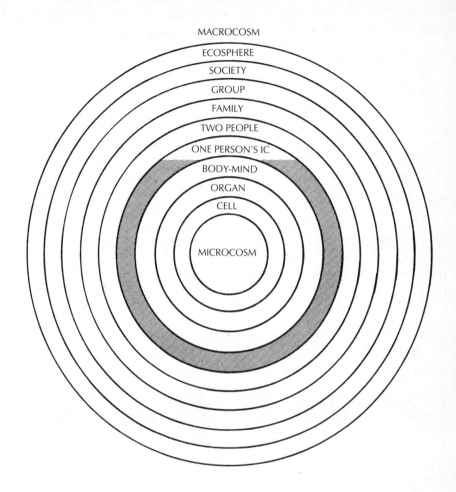

MACROCOSM
ECOSPHERE
SOCIETY
GROUP
FAMILY
TWO PEOPLE
ONE PERSON'S IC
BODY-MIND
ORGAN
CELL

MICROCOSM

Figure 3: Examples of HOLONS

Everything between the macrocosm and microcosm can profitably be viewed as a holon. This means that it is simultaneously a whole in relation to its parts, and a part in relation to the wider whole(s). The microcosm (where quantum physics holds sway) is related to the macrocosm (where relativity holds sway), in that both differ from the human sphere, where the IC attempts to hold sway. The IC does so partly through common sense, which can set many limits, and also through self-transcendence, which can help to override many limits.

the patient's IC, not unlike the way a heart-lung machine takes over for the patient's circulation during open heart surgery. But the essence of both procedures is that they must be temporary.

For Jason it was a big relief to have the doctor making all necessary decisions for a time, taking the blame if something went wrong, and offering Jason the support necessary to "pull himself together."

When Jason gradually succeeded in this effort, part of the self to which he returned was familiar, but part was new growth. This time, the doctor's help was more like crutches, offering security while Jason, in gingerly fashion, tried out his fresh capacities and slowly integrated them into the rest of his unique character.

The uniqueness of the individual starts at conception. In addition to the protein configurations of almost all his cells, there is also the particular arrangement of the cellular "glue" that binds groups of cells together. The special configuration, together with other forms of "marking," enable our cells to spot the unfamiliar ones as nonself.

Without such power of recognition, the immune system could not guard the person against foreign microbes or, some doctors believe, occasional free-floating cancer cells. So thorough is the cellular power of recognition that even a transplant from an identical twin may be rejected as "foreign," even though its cells are genetically the same. (There is some evidence that transplants from a loving and willing donor thrive better than those from a reluctant or unknown one.)

Although one person's cells can readily spot the difference between someone elses and his own, there are times when some of his cells become confused by messages from different parts of himself. For example, inflammatory diseases, such as rheumatoid arthritis, lupus erythematosus, myesthenia gravis, and juvenile-onset diabetes, are believed to derive in part from mixed internal signals about what is self; for some reason, the self's defender cells turn against other of the self's indigenous cells.

Individual cells, in rudimentary form, appear to have not only a will to live but also a capacity for attraction and repulsion, and even a minute ability to learn from experience. Says psychobiologist Myron A. Hofer, "It has only been in the last few years that the relationship of cellular function to behaviors has begun to be understood. New knowledge has opened the way to a view of . . . a common set of principles that can be observed in the behavior of a bacterium as well as a person. Simple animals have been found to have simple versions of characteristics once

thought to be essentially human, such as memory, choice and discrimination."*

A degree of purposefulness is shown both by independent cells, such
as bacteria, and by cells integral to a larger entity. In regard to the latter,
their purposefulness needs to be increasingly orchestrated as the creature
grows in complexity. Mary Midgley, British professor of philosophy, does
not use the term IC, but she refers to the deep human need for something
with the same essential qualities: "Human needs are multiple," she writes.
". . . We have many sorts of good because we have many wants. Yet we
have to make sense of them all somehow by a scheme of priori-
ties. . . . We have to follow the working of that *deep need for unity* which
luckily is to be found at the center of them. People have a natural *wish
and capacity to integrate themselves*, a natural *horror of being totally
fragmented*, which makes possible a constant series of bargains and sacrifices to shape their lives" (italics added). † At the same time, many of
these "bargains and sacrifices" also serve to shape their health.

Each person starts out with certain genetic givens. These include such
factors as race, eye color, and body type, which cannot be changed.
Givens also include factors that, though not wholly fixed, are extremely
difficult to change, the so-called "closed instincts." Midgley points to the
nest-building by weaver birds, a complex series of actions that birds raised
in isolation "know" how to perform. "Such genetic programming," she
writes, "takes the place of intelligence; learning is just maturation. Open
instincts are programs with a gap."

The human is the creature with the greatest number of such "open
instincts." Into their "gaps" come the multitude of individual choices
that need to be coordinated by the person's IC. One instinct that is
"closed" in almost all animals and "open" in humans is sex. Because
the human female does not go into estrus, she is not driven to mate with
the nearest available male, nor he with her, at a set time of the year.
She, therefore, like the man, can use intelligence and other faculties to
choose whether, when, and with whom to mate. Human freedom of
will, in fact, has been traced by some philosophers to this form of biological evolution.

Self-image becomes part of the human IC, but it is not the whole of
it. And some people's self-image is difficult for others to gauge. Many

*Myron A. Hofer, *The Roots of Human Behavior* (New York: Freeman, 1981).
†Mary Midgley, *Beast and Man: The Roots of Human Nature* (Ithaca, N.Y.: Cornell
University Press, 1978).

extremely thin women, for example, nonetheless picture themselves as fat. One individual may be neglecting his dress and hair because a potent IC is elsewhere occupied; Albert Einstein was famous for his unkempt long curls and the lack of one or both of his socks. Yet Dorothy's mother, Martha, a person with low self-image, remained unkempt because she felt too unworthy to allow the hospital nurses to waste their time combing her hair.

Ordinarily, one sign of returning health in chronic mental patients is a new interest in improving their appearance. Yet the typical adolescent who, like a parakeet, cannot pass a mirror without peering long into it, may have an undeveloped and wobbly IC.*

The IC is likely to grow in strength as the person matures. Its typically self-confident operation during later middle age and early old age may have been the reason for Winston Churchill's characterization of these as "the broad sunlit uplands of life." And May Sarton, at seventy, wrote, "I am more myself than I have ever been."

Through experience, the person has learned what is his characteristic style, and, with seeming effortlessness, his IC continues to adjudicate the inevitable conflicts between his three brains and all the other levels of his four dimensions. Says Roger Sperry, M.D., in *Science and Moral Priority: The Merging of Mind, Brain, and Values*, "The whole, besides being different from and greater than the sum of the parts, also causally determines the fate of the parts without interfering with the physical or chemical laws of the sub-entities at their own level."

Though the IC incorporates what Freud called "ego strength," it goes beyond this. For one thing, the IC is connected to all four dimensions, not just to mind and body. For another, it includes a spiritual outreach that Freud denigrated but Jung extolled.† Within the Western tradition, one could say that the individual as a whole—in effect, the IC—is what is "known" by God or by the person to whom one "gives" oneself in love. Within the Eastern tradition, one could say that the unlimited or universal Self (capital S), not the limited or egocentric self (small s), is what the individual needs to focus on. In both traditions, the ensuing

---

*According to a 1984 study by psychologist Joan Harvey of the University of Pennsylvania Medical School, many young high achievers cannot enjoy their success because they feel themselves to be fakes; only in later life do they learn to relax and enjoy, rather than be anxious about, doing better than other people.

†One of the issues on which the Freud-Jung friendship foundered was the role of the spiritual in mental health. While Freud saw human belief in God as wish-fulfillment and regression to infantile dependence on an all-powerful parental figure, Jung saw it as resonating with the most profound aspects of reality and thus providing a stable foundation for good mental health.

experience of merger may include two aspects. The one is reminiscent of what Freud poetically termed the "oceanic feeling"; the other, of what the Gospels inspirationally termed "new life." Today both may be included in psychologist Abraham Maslow's term *peak experience*. Afterward the person feels different and is likely to act differently to such an extent that other people take note of it: "By their fruits shall ye know them."

An historic example was Saint Paul, whose peak experience on the road to Damascus involved the whole of him. His *body* fell to the ground; his *mind* saw a vision; his relationship with *people* radically changed; his *environment* became that of an endangered nomad, and his *IC* was so altered that he insisted people recognize this through calling him by a different name (Paul, rather than Saul).

A contemporary example was Jason's experience in the ocean under the moon. Somehow his IC was emboldened to feel itself integrally related to what really matters. To return to land and proceed with his life, not passively let it be swept under, was part of this mattering.

When Abraham Maslow, in the 1930s, started studying healthy people rather than sick ones, his aim was to discover how they fulfilled their highest potential, thus "actualizing" themselves. This method, he hoped, could then be taught to therapists, who would transmit it to patients and thus put them in touch with their "authentic" spiritual selves.

Since then, peak experiences have been studied in outer space and ocean depths, in young athletes and dying elders. One common characteristic is the memorable quality of the experience. Another is the change that often results from it. Jason, for example, had been trying to tough out his bereavement. He had moved away from as many reminders of his sister as possible, but nothing could give him the slightest pleasure. Symptoms in his *body* then provided an excuse to withdraw from the responsibilities of his work *environment* and his relationship to other people; yet, when his bodily symptoms were alleviated, he felt no relief of *mind*. After his experience in the moonlit ocean, he felt flexible enough to admit his need for professional assistance despite the threat that he feared it might pose to his still-fragile IC.

For many, if not all, people, a peak experience involves the IC's aspect of self-transcendance. As Arthur D. Coleman, M.D., and Libby Lee Coleman write in *Love and Ecstasy*, "Ecstatic journeys tend to follow a certain order, as if the brain has only a few stereotyped paths with which to order an 'I-less' world: The experience of merger is a sweeping transformation of our ordinary frame of reality."

One such transformation is evoked by psychologist Ira Progoff in *The Well and the Cathedral*. As people go down deeper into the well of self, he says, the lucky ones reach all the way to the subterranean spring that nourishes every individual well. Truly to know that at the profoundest level of communication *there are no strangers* may provide a faltering IC with the additional strength it needs.

This form of wisdom, however, is not new. The playwright Terence, in ancient Rome, noted that "nothing human is alien to me." What *is* new is to conceptualize IC wholeness as analagous to the lensless photography called *holography*. First a wave field of light is scattered by the chosen object. Then the picture is recorded, partly directly, partly by way of a semisilvered mirror. In ordinary light, the resulting film appears only as a mass of meaningless snowy swirls, but if you shine a laser beam on it, a three-dimensional representation emerges that is so vivid that someone looking at it might mistake it for the real object. Spookiest of all, if you tear up the film and shine a laser beam on a tiny part of it, the *whole picture* reappears.

Some scientists, such as Stanford University neuroscientist Karl Pribram, conjecture that the human brain operates in a holographic manner. How else to explain the way huge segments can be injured without the personality being altered? Presidential press secretary James Brady, shot with President Reagan on March 30, 1981, had so much of his brain damaged that some doctors predicted he would die; others said that if he survived, he would be little better than a vegetable. Yet Brady's IC will-to-live and sense of humor never deserted him. Also significant to his extraordinary recovery was the daily presence of his wife and daughter, who kept telling him things to make him smile—and later tossing a bean bag with him.

A contrasting example of a whole life clouded by one confidence-shattering remark was reported by Lillian Hellman in *Maybe*. An early lover had accused her of having "female odor." Here was her *body* impinging on her relationship with *people*, with devastating results for her *mind*. She subsequently refused to live in any *environment* without a tub, and took at least three baths daily. Even so, with subsequent lovers, she was apprehensive. Only much later did her determination (IC), to discover all the facts of the case free her from this burden. After talking to other women who had known her early lover, she learned that he had made the same sadistic remark to them. That was *his* characteristic pattern, and once she was aware of it as such, she could extricate herself from its baneful effects.

As Jerome Kagan, professor of developmental psychology at Harvard, puts it, "Emotional states can be altered through information." On the other hand, as many patients in psychotherapy complain, *knowing* something and *feeling* it can be two very different experiences.

An example of an IC that enabled a person to rise above agonizing feelings based on deprivation is that of Helen Keller. Rendered totally blind and deaf by a fever when she was a happy, healthy nineteen months of age, she became enraged (mind), hyperactive (body), a torment to her family (other people), and a destroyer of her possessions (environment). Her immature IC had been overwhelmed. But Anne Sullivan, a teacher who, in her own girlhood, had overcome serious physical, emotional, and financial deprivation, was finally able to establish dialogue with Helen by spelling words into her palm. No longer were Helen's blindness and deafness a total prison. She pulled herself together (IC), and went on to become an inspiring leader. Having finally made peace with reality, she showed herself to be a basically healthy person who was missing two capacities, rather than what she had been before, a fragmented and unhealthy person. On the other hand, her childish tantrums may have been a signal that a strong IC was there to be tapped, having presumably developed during her wholesome first almost-two-years of life.

The perennial question of why suffering diminishes some people and ennobles or invigorates others has had new light cast on it by a working group at the Hastings Institute of Society, Ethics, and the Life Sciences. Their conclusion was to distinguish between *pain*, on the one hand, and *suffering*, on the other.* The report, written by Eric J. Cassel, M.D., professor of public health at Cornell Medical School, maintains, in effect, that *pain* can be felt in any of the four dimensions, but *suffering* is a function of the IC. As Cassel sums it up, "Suffering is experienced by persons, not merely by bodies, and has its source in challenges that threaten the intactness of the person as a complex social and psychological entity." Doctors, moreover, by failing to understand the difference between pain and suffering, often take technical steps to cure the pain, steps that increase the suffering.

One example is the treatment of childbirth in old-fashioned American hospitals. Obstetricians, without consulting the patient, administer analgesics that blunt the pain but muddle the woman's sense of self, thus leaving her with no center from which to cope with the predictably recurring pain, and thereby increasing her suffering.

Individuals vary greatly in their threshold of pain as well as their willingness to undergo it for the sake of a higher aim.† No matter how painful giving birth may have been the first time, most women are willing

---

*Eric J. Cassel, "The Nature of Suffering and the Goals of Medicine," New England Journal of Medicine, 18 March 1982.
†Some individuals, according to psychologist J. Peter Rosenfeld, can decrease their sensitivity to pain by learning through biofeedback to control the kind of brainwave called EP or evoked potential (Mary Travis, "Pain and the Brain," Psychology Today, December, 1984).

to go through it again, and martyrs have staked out the far pole of pain in order to feel closer to God's will; though tortured, their feeling was presumably less one of suffering than of purpose fulfilled.

Similarly, a sense of triumph may result from the IC's battling of an illness. Marvella Bayh, wife of former senator Birch Bayh of Indiana, rose to new spiritual and interpersonal heights in the years between the discovery of her breast cancer and her death. At first she was in despair. She was only in early middle age, her son was still very young, and her husband's career, in which she played a substantive part, was still in need of her assistance. But the more she learned about how the individual, with the help of chosen doctors, can retard the growth of cancer, and the more she wrote and lectured about it, the more her readers' and audiences' gratitude ricocheted healthfully back onto her. As she wrote in her autobiography, "These years"—which were many more than the doctors had predicted—"have been the most rewarding, the most fulfilling, the happiest of my life."*

Whatever serves to strengthen the patient probably does so by directly or indirectly engaging his IC. Some people try "positive *thinking*": They count their blessings. Others try "positive *feeling*": They develop what family therapist Virginia Satir calls "an appreciation of themselves; that doesn't mean showing off—feeling good about yourself isn't the same as saying I'm better than you—it means being enthusiastic about life."†

In a comparison of people who succumbed to serious stress and those who not only survived it but, to a degree, enjoyed it, University of Chicago researcher Suzanne C. Kobasa studied several hundred executives at Illinois Bell Telephone Company. While the stress *victims* characteristically viewed change as an unwelcome disruption, the stress *managers* viewed it as a welcome opportunity in which they could maintain some degree of control. The stress managers, furthermore, sensed within themselves a strong sense of purpose: Whatever the change, it was not going to lick them; *they* were going to harness *it*. The victims, in contrast, felt themselves at the mercy of unpredictable developments.

Some people master stress by mobilizing one of their so-called negative feelings, such as anger or aggression. Said philosopher George Santayana, "To knock a thing down, especially if it is cocked at an arrogant angle, is a deep delight to the blood."

Still others move outward in objectivity as well as inward in subjectivity.

---

*Marvella Bayh and Mary L. Kotz, *Marvella: A Personal Journey* (San Diego: Harcourt Brace Jovanovich, 1981).
†Some psychologically oriented surgeons refuse to perform an elective operation on a patient who seems too thoroughly pessimistic about life in general and this operation in particular.

Theirs is a deliberate bifocal perspective. An example is the patient who, on receiving news of her grave ailment, asked, "Why me?" But then, rising above the situation, she asked, "Why not me?" and finally focused on the responsible question "What am I going to do about it?"*

What one chooses to do about a serious health—or other—problem depends in part on one's value system. For Freud, an atheist, there was reference to something akin to the IC: "In the small decisions of life," he wrote, "I call upon my judgment; in the large ones I follow my unconscious."

For religious people, such as Rabbi Harold S. Kushner, there is prayer: "One of the things that constantly reassures me that God is real, and not just an idea that religious leaders made up, is the fact that people who pray for strength, hope, and courage so often find resources of strength, hope, and courage that they did not have before they prayed."†

For other people, such as columnist Stewart Alsop (author of *Stay of Execution*), there is the unconscious defense of humor. "Uncle Thanatos" was Alsop's nickname for the Grim Reaper, against whom he did manful battle while postponing for many years his predicted death from leukemia. As theologian Reinhold Niebuhr pointed out, humor and prayer are alike, in that both attempt to deal creatively with life's worst incongruities.

Both humor and prayer were put to use by writer Flannery O'Connor. With the help of her mother, she postponed death from lupus erythematosus for many years. As Alsop did, she sublimated part of her suffering into memorable prose. In one of her letters (in *The Habit of Being*), she wrote: "I have never been anywhere but sick. In a sense sickness is a place, more instructive than a long trip to Europe. . . . Sickness before death is a very appropriate thing and I think those who don't have it miss one of God's mercies. . . . I come from a family where the only emotion respectable to show is irritation. In some this tendency produces hives, in others, literature, in me both."

Indeed, all the arts, as well as crafts, may provide their practitioner, amateur as well as professional, with a valuable method of organizing reality. This, in turn, may result in a sense of mastery that boosts the IC. When novelist Anthony Burgess was told in 1959 that his newly discovered tumor would kill him within the year, he sat down and wrote

---

*Many men who went on to become president had a far worse-than-average medical history, as with Lincoln's severe depressions, Theodore Roosevelt's asthma and tuberculosis, Woodrow Wilson's history of apparent strokes, Franklin D. Roosevelt's polio, John F. Kennedy's Addison's disease and injured spine, and Lyndon B. Johnson's serious heart attack. Yet these men, it is clear, also had better-than-average stick-to-it-iveness.
†Harold S. Kushner, *When Bad Things Happen to Good People* (New York: Schocken Books, 1981).

five novels in that time; now, twenty-five years later, he is alive and well and writing in England.

In regard to Jason, quitting his guitar playing, though understandable in terms of his lethargy, was probably counterproductive in terms of his IC. In contrast, Meritt B. Low, M.D., who was felled by polio, struggled forcefully to live a rich life despite his sharply limited capacities: "The personality affects the disease more than the disease affects the personality," he writes. "It isn't the condition itself but the view one takes of it that is the real crux."

Doctors can often greatly help a patient by trying to understand and reinforce his particular approach to life. In his autobiographical A *Leg to Stand On*, neurologist Oliver Sacks, of Albert Einstein College of Medicine, writes about his hospital experiences in England as both patient and doctor: "What I felt so intensely . . . was a need to assert and affirm the living subject, to escape from a purely objective . . . science, to find and establish what was mising—a living 'I.' "

JUNE: Why do you want people more aware of their IC?

NORMAN: So they can look inward, analyze what's going on in their four
             dimensions, and mobilize the IC to break into a vicious cycle
             within or between these before it gains too much momentum.

JUNE: Can the IC collapse from that kind of effort?

NORMAN: Not really. Or not for long. The essence of the individual
             remains. People sometimes fear therapy because they think it
             will make them lose themselves in some fundamental way.
             But the only time that kind of thing happens is under the
             influence of powerful mind-altering drugs, like LSD, or pro-
             longed torture.

JUNE: What about people whose IC is deranged by alcohol?

NORMAN: I personally don't believe that alcohol or most drugs are ever
             a full excuse for anyone's behavior. Sure, they release inhi-
             bitions enough for people to say or do things they are usually
             too cautious to. But most people, under most circumstances,
             are aware of what they're doing. We can be provoked, but how
             we respond to that provocation is partially under our control.
             In the Roman Catholic doctrine, even the people considered
             to be possessed by the devil are assumed to retain an element
             of free will. The main point is for people to have faith in their
             own IC and realize that it's indelible and has survival value.

JUNE: And health value?

NORMAN: Very much so. More, I expect, than any of the dimensions by itself.

JUNE: What about people who have a problem in some dimension, and all that their IC can come up with is self-pity?

NORMAN: Well, at first self-pity may be an appropriate reaction, especially if the blow has been severe; but if the self-pity continues for too long, it may turn off other people. It may also use up energy that is better put to experimenting with active ways to improve the situation.

JUNE: Maybe that's what happened with Job. He started with self-pity, and at first his three friends were sympathetic; but then they turned against him, saying he must have sinned terribly to have brought such disasters on himself.

NORMAN: People still love to lay guilt on an invalid.

JUNE: Then Job got mad. His IC rallied. He was able to move out beyond his poor old body riddled with boils, and his poor old mind mourning for all his dead children and lost possessions.

NORMAN: The IC stretched his perspective.

JUNE: Then Job lifted up his eyes and marveled at the heavens. In comparison with the wonders of the universe, he said, his own sufferings, even those of all humankind, were as nothing.

NORMAN: Job rose above his situation through awe; Norman Cousins and Stewart Alsop rose above theirs through laughter.

JUNE: And Jason? Did he rise above his through some medication?

NORMAN: Not at all! When the doctor figures that the target organ is the IC, then the last thing he wants is to dull the patient's perceptions. He wants the patient to study his own dimensions carefully and try to spot which of his patterns are combining in an unwholesome manner.

JUNE: And Jason did that?

NORMAN: With the help of his doctor, he took inventory. When his sister died, this pushed his button, his old unresolved conflict over his mother's death when he was eight. At the time, he was told to be a big boy and not cry. He never discussed with anyone the depth of his sorrow, nor did he let himself realize the terrible rage he felt at *her* for deserting him. As the years passed, he forgot all about these feelings, but when his sister became terminally ill, his helplessness to do anything for her, combined with his grief, made him half-crazy. Abruptly, he moved across town; but then he did nothing to settle himself or get to know his neighbors—or even find out where the dry cleaner was. Some people seem born with a strong, resilient IC. The more bad things that happen to them, the more challenged they feel. They roll with the punches—or they fight back.

JUNE: But Jason didn't fight. He fled.

NORMAN: In a sense, he also went limp. He became passive.

JUNE: Is that an IC function, to choose which of the coping mechanisms to use?

NORMAN: At an unconscious level, I think it is. What Jason needed to do was get busy with what Freud had called "the work of grief." And it *is* work, especially when, like one of the neurochemicals, bereavement binds itself to a previously sensitized emotional "receptor area."

JUNE: Such as?

NORMAN: Such as Jason's childhood rage at being both helpless and vulnerable when his mother died. To deal with death, even as an adult, is to face one's ultimate helplessness. For Jason as an adult, there was a further unresolved conflict between his desolation at his sister's death and his relief that at last he was free to grow up and be independent. He also felt a common form of relief in that if *someone* in the family had to die, it wasn't himself.

JUNE: Is that part of survivor guilt?

NORMAN: In part. Germans call it *Schadenfreude*. You've seen people smile in spite of themselves when they give—or receive—bad news. It's not the most admirable aspect of human nature, but it reflects a healthy IC's will to live.

JUNE: What about Jason?

NORMAN: His IC might have had a geological "fault," like California's San Andreas Fault. No matter how carefully he supervised his health, when an area close to the "fault" shifted, a fissure opened up in his health. His will to live wasn't all that strong. He needed help in keeping the whole thing "together." That may be why he swam so far out in the ocean.

JUNE: Like Keats's "I am half in love with easeful death"?

NORMAN: Jason was more than half. Some people deliberately keep flirting with death. They take crazy short-term risks to titillate their IC's exultance in being alive, or they indulge in long-term self-destructive habits, such as smoking or drinking too much. These mask themselves as pleasure, but underneath, like Mary Ellen's failed suicide attempt, they may be an unconscious attempt to get help.

JUNE: Is that what Freud meant by the death wish?

NORMAN: Freud suggested that what we call self-preservation may simply be the organism's desire to die at its own time, in its own fashion. Since Freud's day, biologists have found that our cells and organs are genetically programmed to self-destruct when their appointed season arrives. So Thanatos, and the death wish, can be seen as necessary to ecological, as well as individual, health. If your old blood cells didn't die off and make room for new ones, your general health would suffer. And imagine if all the people ever born were still hanging around!

JUNE: Yet, given their choice, a lot of them *would* be.

NORMAN: I don't doubt it. Some very old people, with all their functions gravely impaired, struggle to stay alive, no matter what. Others don't wish to live in any such condition. For example, Christiaan Barnard, the famous heart surgeon, has a pact with his doctor brother that if either of them seriously loses his mental powers, the other will actively help end his life.

JUNE: Is that an example of the IC being strong?

NORMAN: I think so. Some people care more about quality of life than quantity; others care more about quantity. The main thing is for the person's IC not to wind down ahead of his four dimensions.

JUNE: You mean, like the one-hoss-shay, with all four wheels and axles collapsing at the same time?

NORMAN: That one-hoss-shay must have had a marvelous IC.

VIII
Grounds for a Healthy Scepticism

Final Report on Mary Ellen and Jason

"The older I grow, the more impressed I am with the role of luck or chance in life."
—Sidney Hook (in his eighties)

The day after Mary Ellen crossed the street in order to avoid Jason, she was forced to see him at their therapy group. Afterward, with the doctor's permission, they went out for coffee. He told her about his brush with suicide. He spoke with wonder at Nancy and Bill's affection, especially when he had spiraled down into so obnoxious a form of depression.

Mary Ellen was lifted out of her self-absorption by his honesty. She admired his courage in facing up to the unflattering aspect of his emotions. Only someone who had gone down to the depths of self-hatred, she felt, could understand her own constant self-doubting. With her slowly developing trust in him came a crumbling of inner barriers against her yearning to love.

Her gentle dependence made Jason feel ten feet tall. After a year of dating, Mary Ellen brought Jason home for her parents to meet. Her mother's unfeigned joy in Mary Ellen's happiness made Mary Ellen forgive her for the past. Her father, too, was impressed with Jason, and the two men contentedly spent hours together.

Jason was the first to terminate treatment. Finally, Mary Ellen, too, was ready. They got married. On their second anniversary they decided to start a family. A couple of months later they went to join Bill and Nancy at the beach. On the plane, Mary Ellen sat next to a

ten-year-old boy and played checkers on a tiny magnetic board he
had brought along.

Not long after their return home, Mary Ellen felt blah for a day
and her complexion was blotched, but by the next morning, all was
well again. She never thought to mention the episode to Jason, nor
to the obstetrician whom she began visiting when she suspected she
was pregnant. Half a year later she gave birth to a handsome son.
But he had no startle reaction to sudden noise. He was deaf.

When the pediatrician gave her the bad news, Mary Ellen began
to weep, and could not stop. Jason kept trying to console her, but
his words had no impact. The baby's deafness, she insisted, must be
a judgment upon her. She shouldn't have drunk that one glass of
champagne on New Year's Eve; she should have given up coffee
completely; above all, she and Jason shouldn't have slept together
before marriage.

Jason called their priest. The priest came and assured Mary Ellen
that God's ways are mysterious to man, but that in His plan, all things
come right in the end. He prayed by her bedside and reminded her
that God's forgiveness extends to *all* his children.

She continued to weep.

Jason called their psychiatrist. He came and explained that temporary hormonal imbalance causes many a new mother to suffer from
postpartum (postbirth) sadness and tears. He assured her she would
soon feel more normal and prescribed a mild tranquilizer, which she
refused to take. She was nursing the baby and feared that the drug
might come through in the milk.

She continued to weep.

Frantic, Jason queried the obstetrician about all possible causes
for the baby's disability. One was German measles (rubella), especially when contracted during the first trimester of pregnancy. With
the help of the airline, Jason found the address of the boy who had
sat next to them. Jason phoned his parents. Yes, the boy had come
down with German measles the day after arrival at the beach.

Jason sat at the edge of Mary Ellen's bed and took her hand. He
pointed out the plain bad luck they had suffered; first in the flight
they had chosen, then in her sitting next to the imminently sick boy.
In addition to the separate randomness of these events, there was the
random way they had occurred at the specific time when the fetus
was most vulnerable to damage by that virus.

She continued to weep.

Jason lost control.

"Don't keep wallowing in some goddamn imaginary sin!" he

shouted. "There was nothing you could have done. Let's start thinking about what we're going to do now."

Shocked, she stared at him. He had never spoken to her like that. Her tears dried. Having a deaf child was bad enough. But having a deaf child whose parents were divorced would be worse. Gingerly she took his hand. "Just because our baby's deaf," she said, "you don't need to yell."

Scientific knowledge, as the late Warren Weaver, said, is like a clearing in an impenetrable forest. The wider the circumference of the known, the greater the contact with the unknown.

A healthy scepticism, therefore, should be part of the individual's response whenever people try to impose on him some newly minted panacea or simplistic health warning in terms that arouse anxiety. Recommended as a corrective is the kind of open-ended thinking exemplified by Dr. Lewis Thomas's in an informal speech given to the staff of Memorial Sloan Kettering Hospital in New York. After agreeing that 80 percent of cancers in humans are caused by environmental factors, Dr. Thomas suggested that this claim be "interpreted rather differently from the way it is commonly perceived. It is based on observable differences in this or that . . . society, that is, how many more stomach cancers we have here than they have there, and so forth. The assumption is made that maybe in each of those . . . communities there is something special in the environment, or in the diet . . . that causes that kind of cancer. . . .

"The trouble . . . is that in each of the societies observed, the *overall* incidence of cancer is *not very different.* . . . There has to be *something else going on* . . . that we don't understand" (italics added). *

Something else *is* going on, not merely in regard to the disease being studied, but also, often, within the people who collect the statistics and those who apply them. More goes on than meets the software of even the best computer terminal.

Since computers can do only what human beings tell them, and since human beings, including scientists, are subject to their own unconscious desires and fears, many a researcher may simply *fail to notice* some factor that would complicate, if not jeopardize, his hypothesis. As with the difference between people who describe a glass as half-full and those who say it is half-empty, much depends on who is doing the estimating

*This speech was reprinted in the *Cancer Center Bulletin*, Winter 1979.

and why. As John Stuart Mill wrote, "The seer changes what is seen."*

As for the person trying to decide whether a particular set of health statistics applies to himself, much depends on his heredity, environments, and attitude, the approach of his doctor or other helping person, and the many other forms of "something else" that causally or randomly are "going on" at that particular time.

If, for example, a bookie had been asked for odds beforehand on Mary Ellen's bearing a deaf child, he would have set them extremely low. Yet that is what occurred because of the random event of her sitting next to a sick boy on a plane ride.

On the other hand, a happy example of bucking the causal odds was Winston Churchill. Born of a beautiful mother who either ignored him or acted seductively, and a brilliant, severe father who went insane, Churchill remained in good enough mental health to serve successfully in several hugely stressful positions and live on into his nineties despite having consumed sides of marbled beef, mountains of puddings, cases of brandy and champagne, smoking shiploads of cigars, keeping very late hours, and studiously avoiding exercise. From early manhood, however, he had had the support of a loyal and understanding wife.

In the United States, alarming health statistics are often blazoned in the media. Sometimes the motive for such publicity is openly to sell a product; other times, the motive may be disguised. Not long ago, public suspicion was aroused that a series of magazine articles decrying the harmful effects of stress had been commissioned by a manufacturer of tranquilizers.

In regard to the newest so-called miracle drug, as well as the newest prediction of health damage, therefore, the consumer does well to apply the old first rule for journalists, to establish promptly "who, what, when, where," as well as "why." The consumer should also bear in mind that the United States is probably the most fad-prone of all countries. Not long ago, eggs were the big no-no; now eggs are being recommended in moderation because several of their essential nutrients are harder to come upon elsewhere. Mary Ellen's assumption that her one glass of champagne on New Year's Eve could have caused the baby's deafness was subjectively understandable but objectively false. Common sense rather than Spartan absolutism is, in general, the best policy for pregnancy and other stressful stages.

*After Mill's day, scientific proof of alteration of the seen by the seer was provided by Einstein's theory of relativity in the macrocosm, and Heisenberg's principle of uncertainty in the microcosm.

Even when the statistics are correct and the person finds himself in an endangered category, he need not despair. Suppose the incidence of flu is burgeoning in his locale. The prediction is that one person in three will sicken. Individual A is frightened but does nothing; Individual B is certain he will stay well and does nothing; Individual C is alarmed enough to get a flu shot. No doctor can say for sure which two out of the three will escape the flu, for so much depends on the individual's four dimensions and IC and whether these are acting in harmony at the time or not. For instance:

- In the realm of *body*, did the flu he had last year leave him with adequate antibodies?
- In the realm of *mind*, is he able to relax at times or does he constantly feel driven?
- In the realm of *environments*, does he take a crowded subway every day or live isolated in the country?
- In the realm of *other people*, is he living only with adults or with a small child whose only form of learning at nursery school, it seems, is how to come home with a different disease each week? In the former instance, do the adults tend to "punish" him for his continued good health by loading too many responsibilities on him, or by taking his efforts too much for granted?
- In the realm of the *IC*, is he at a stage when, because of the nature of his work or responsibilities, he really does not want to get sick and therefore, in many instances, does not? Or was he formerly in that stage, and is now no longer?

When a person falls seriously ill, an important, though from his point of view accidental, factor in his recovery may be the attitude of his doctor that day. How is the doctor feeling toward this patient as an individual? Toward this type of illness as potentially curable? Toward himself as a trustworthy conveyor of cure in this type of case?

Often, if the patient has sufficient faith in the doctor, the latter can prescribe a placebo (a neutral substance) as if it were a medication, and the patient's symptoms will promptly disappear. Evidence is accumulating that being given a supposedly healing substance increases the person's production of certain hormones, perhaps even essential neurochemicals.

Today, the term placebo effect has expanded, according to Harvard's Herbert Benson, M.D., to include all nonspecific aspects of treatment, including, in addition to the attitude of the doctor, the type of setting in which treatment takes place. "Under certain circumstances," Dr. Benson writes, "placebos have alleviated pain, healed ulcers, improved the electrocardiogram, and enhanced exercise performances. They have also provided relief from hay fever, coughing, and hypertension."

In brain research, if a heroin addict has already been given a shot of nalaxone (an opiate antagonist), his later heroin injection will have no effect. The same thing happens to people known to be responsive to placebos: A previous shot of nalaxone prevents the *placebo* from having an effect. This suggests a physical basis for the placebo effect, one that perhaps stimulates the brain to produce more endorphins. Further evidence for this physical component is the fixed proportion of people (around a third) who respond to placebos in a positive manner, regardless of race or sex, age or geography.

In addition to the positive placebo effect, there is also a negative one (nocebo). If a patient is warned that the substance being given him is harmful, he may develop a headache, rash, heart palpitation, or intestinal upset. The worst kind of negative placebo would presumably be the witch doctor capable of putting the "evil eye" on someone, or sticking pins into his effigy, until he sickens and dies.*

What the evil eye can do in a primitive culture, an alarming health statistic may do in a post-industrial one. If I read that my age-group, or sex, or race, is prone to a certain disease, I may feel jinxed. I may need reassurance—perhaps partly placebo effect—from a doctor or other authority-figure who says, "*You* don't need to worry about that."

Patients pick up so easily on their doctor's expectation for them that the testing of new drugs is thereby skewed. As a result, the "double blind" experiment had to be devised: In addition to the patient remaining unaware of whether he is getting a real medication or a placebo, the administering person also must be unaware.

Yet even when a placebo is administered by a stranger—or a machine—it may have benign effects. For example, a group of schizophrenic patients were given renal dialysis, a form of blood-cleansing by a machine performing as a kidney. A control group, matched as to age and sex, degree and duration of illness, were not. The first group began behaving in a much more rational manner. Could some harmful chemical really have been removed from their blood? But, no, their blood chemistry was little different from the control group's; the benefit appeared to come from having been given so much attention by machine, as well as by people, within an atmosphere of hope for improvement.

Some medical tools are so potent and specific that the most disinterested, even hostile, technician can spur healing—say, by administering insulin to a diabetic, vitamin D to a child with rickets, or morphine to

*The killing power of the witch doctor is believed to derive in part from his ability to mobilize the three primal fears of humankind, namely, of death, mutilation, and being cast out by one's group.

a patient in agony. Patient expectations are also so potent that preoperative people who are shown a videotape about what to expect—and as a result are not later subjected to unpleasant surprises—end up needing less anesthesia during the operation, fewer painkillers afterward, and tend to heal faster than matched patients who do not see the videotape. Some patients also respond well to wholesome suggestions made during hypnosis or at the time of emergence from anesthesia.

Even under deep anesthesia, some patients have been observed to pick up negative expectations voiced by their surgeon. Sometimes, in fact, these turn into a form of "self-fulfilling prophecy." In one instance, a woman with bowel cancer, though thoroughly anesthetized, may have heard her surgeon tell the interns, "This case won't live more than two years." Later on, to her, he said that he had "gotten it all" and she should go home and enjoy a normal life. This she did, feeling well and gaining needed weight. But exactly two years later she asked to be admitted to the hospital. Her symptoms were vague; all she could say was that she felt too ill to cope. She soon died. On autopsy, she was found to be free of cancer. Subsequent hypnosis of the interns from two years before brought recall of the surgeon's prediction. No other reason for her death could be found.

Psychologist Henry Bennett, of the University of California at Davis, reports on a plump woman whose surgeon said, after she had been fully anesthetized, "My God, they've dragged another beached whale onto my operating table." During her postoperative period, the patient was plagued with various problems, including fever. Suddenly, a week later, the insulting memory surfaced and she complained to a nurse, who verified it. Within twelve hours the patient felt well enough to go home. How well her surgeon felt when she confronted him is not reported.*

So strong is human suggestibility that medical students often suffer, in turn, the symptoms of whatever ailment they are studying. They soon learn, however, not to take these temporary, though genuine, pains too seriously. The awareness that their colleagues are similarly afflicted also helps to alleviate their anxiety.

But the ordinary citizen is not similarly forewarned, nor does he necessarily have nearby colleagues with whom to compare notes when dire warnings appear against such ordinary activities as:
• occasionally eating cheese (animal fat; *body*)
• reacting passively to serious loss (*mind*)
• being deserted through death or divorce (*other people*)
• spending time on, or even near, a highway (*environments*)

*Kevin McKean, "In Search of the Unconscious Mind," *Discover*, February 1985.

• becoming so confused by the plethora of warnings that he despairs of ever achieving or retaining good health (IC)

Whenever one feels unduly apprehensive because of some health statistic, it is worth recalling that in the worst of history's recorded epidemics, Europe's Black Plague in the fourteenth century, only half the populace died; *the other half survived.* Some lucky people must not have caught the disease; some must have caught it and recovered; and some must have had what today would be termed a *subclinical case.* This type of case is not detectable except by vague symptoms (like Mary Ellen's rubella) and modern blood tests but is still sufficient to elicit the antibodies that conquer the germs and provide later immunity.

In short, just because an individual belongs in a high-risk category does not mean that all dire predictions are going to apply, especially when he enjoys some aspect of his life and can mobilize some free-will aspect of his IC on behalf of improving his health.

Whether free will exists *objectively* has long been debated, with no philosopher or scientist able to prove or disprove it.* But *subjectively,* some IC sense that "I am the master of my fate; I am the captain of my soul," may contribute not only to good health but also happiness.

The opposite of feeling self-responsible may be a conviction of helplessness and hopelessness (copelessness). "I'm a poor lorn creature," says a minor character in *David Copperfield,* "and everything goes contrairy with me." And everything did. Today some scientists think there is a connection between this kind of extreme passivity and the unwillingness to fight even against a life-threatening illness, including cancer. Caroline Bedell Thomas, M.D., of Johns Hopkins, for example, started studying 1,337 medical students in 1945 in an attempt to find precursors to heart attack, hypertension, mental ills, suicide, and cancer. She was surprised that the psychological profiles of many subsequent cancer patients were similar to those of suicides. Some of the people in these two categories had perhaps not been born with, or managed to develop, a sturdy IC.

Fortunately, in most of the people, most of the time, most of the diseases go away on their own—or with an assist by the doctor and the patient's IC. This appears to be true of many ailments associated with a particular stage in life.

Some stages end with a bang, others with a whimper. Birth, the abrupt ending of life in utero, is the most dramatic, except for sudden death. The gradual ending of childhood, with the dropping of a boy's voice or

---

*Sir Isaiah Berlin approvingly quotes his fellow philosopher, John Austin: "They all *talk* about determinism and *say* they believe in it. I've never met a determinist in my life, I mean a man who really did believe in it as you and I believe that men are mortal."

the lifting of a girl's breasts, is manifest even to strangers. So, too, may be the years of midlife crisis, for men as well as women, when the waist may thicken and the behavior go off on a tangent. But once the person works through the "passage" to the next stage, he may find a plateau of good health, free from the typical ailments of the previous stage, and not yet subject to the woes of passage to the next one. Distressing conditions, like those listed below, are often simply and gratefully outgrown:

• the recurrent colic that appears in newborns
• the acute panic at the departure of a parental figure ("separation anxiety") that appears in dramatic form between the ages of six months and eighteen months
• the hyperactivity that appears in some young children
• the acne and overweight that appear in some adolescents
• the depression that appears in some young adults, especially between ages twenty-five and forty-four
• the uncharacteristically dramatic mood swings that appear in some men as well as women during the midlife years
• the debility, arthritis, diabetes, and memory loss that appear in some elderly people. Although these forms of woe may not be outgrown, they are more amenable to treatment than used to be assumed. Many bedridden, supposedly senile patients have responded so well to antidepressant drugs and improved nutrition that they arose from their beds and again took part in ordinary life.

Regardless of when in one's life an ailment strikes, much depends on whether the patient's IC characteristically responds with fight, flight, or lying low. Sometimes one of these reactions is the most suitable; sometimes another. Ideally, the IC should be resilient enough to vary its response according to the exigencies of that particular disease. An element of luck, moreover, may enter the health equation in the form of a match between that year's form of ailment and the individual's characteristic coping mechanism.

People who *lie low* may feel and act temporarily helpless, their regression being to either their personal childhood or an evolutionary lizardhood. For them, an interval of handing over responsibility to someone else may be "just what the doctor ordered." Soon they feel the better for the respite. But others make insufficient effort to "get back on their feet" and may need family members or the doctor to force them to bestir themselves.

People who try to *flee* their illness may use the unconscious defense of denial. "I'm *not* getting a cold," they tell themselves as symptoms begin. And sometimes, in fact, the symptoms disappear. But other times the cold may develop and be the worse for having been neglected in its early stages. Denial is also useful (by refusing to look in the mirror) when a face is ravaged by age or injury.

People who *fight* their illness may turn feisty and battle not only their symptoms but also the people taking care of them. This can be hard on the latter but good for the patient. In August 1984, the American Psychological Association was presented with three studies of 232 patients with skin or breast cancer. Those patients who were listless or silently hostile had more recurrence—and died earlier—than those who let their emotions fly.* These observations fitted with a previous Johns Hopkins study of 35 women with advanced breast cancer: those who responded to news of their situation with anger (together with guilt, anxiety, even depression) lived longer, on the average, than those whose attitude was one of copelessness. The angry ones were also described by their doctor as exhibiting what he called "negative attitudes."

Just as the word *accident* needs to be redefined, so does the word *negative* as applied to attitude, for there are times when feelings of hatred or rage can be "positive" through galvanizing a healing fight response. Anger, moreover, as Konrad Lorenz pointed out in his book *On Aggression*, arises only in those species that are also capable of love (love and hate not being each other's true opposites, but indifference being the opposite of them both).

"Negative" sometimes turns out to be "positive" in the laboratory as well as the sickroom. Many a failed or "negative" experiment, when studied, has pointed the way to subsequent ones that yielded the desired result. In the sickroom, if the patient studies an attitude of his own that appears counterproductive, he, too, can try one that may be more successful.

For example, the person who characteristically handles his pain with stoicism and receives little attention from the nurses may find that an occasional loud yelp works better. Similarly, a nonstop complainer may find that forcing himself to express an interest in how someone else is feeling, including his doctor or nurse, works better. Being a successful patient, like other skills, may take practice.

Mary Ellen needed help in learning not only how to be a more successful patient but also how to be a more successful significant other (SO) to that other patient, her newborn son. First she needed to recognize that his bad luck in being born deaf was precisely that: bad luck. Then

*Among the researchers were Sandra Levy of the University of Pittsburgh and Ronald Casey of Yale.

she needed, for his sake and Jason's as well as her own, to break out of her first automatic response, which was to return to the copelessness that had signaled her earlier depression.

Severe depression affects young people more than their elders; so does schizophrenia (the former name of which, *dementia praecox*, reflected this precocity of onset). Thus, while older people have more coexisting chronic physical ailments, they may avoid the worst of the mental ones, unless, of course, Alzheimer's disease takes its terrible toll or a stroke erodes the personality.

In the United States, people alive today are luckier than any large group of Americans has ever been. Since the turn of the century, life expectancy at birth has risen from an average of 47 to 74.6 years, and the quality of life, too, has dramatically improved. For the first time in history, trim, fiber-filled, bright-eyed men and women in their seventies, even eighties, are striding along—or jogging or biking or dancing—in comfortable clothes, appearing more fit than did their grandparents (in corset or stiff collar) in their forties. These people are obviously lucky, not only in their personal circumstances, but also in the medical advances made during their lifetime. * Although eventually these "youthful elderly" will die of the same heart attack, stroke, or cancer that claimed their grandparents, this will occur at a later age. Charles F. Longino, M.D., director of the Center for Social Research in Aging at the University of Miami, has coined the term *youth creep* for the way many current survivors seem young for their advanced age. Though the careers of these people are almost, if not completely, over and their options are reduced, many of them feel as if in wartime: in danger, with every minute counting. By necessity, they have become *now* people, gratefully savoring each pain-free day, even hour.

Not atypical was a mid-1980s obituary that read "Friedy Becker-Wegeli, a still-life artist who *began* her career at the age of 79 while recuperating from a *heart attack*, died . . . at 84. . . . After receiving a pacemaker implant in 1978, she began taking art lessons. . . . Recently she had heard that one of her floral paintings would be accepted for the White House collection . . ." (italics added).

Typical of elderly people is that their diseases are likely to be multiple and their symptoms vague. Sometimes their physician is hard put to figure out why they have simply "taken to their bed." One group of six such patients in their eighties were visibly afflicted by shakiness, mental

---

*There appears to be an inverse relationship between American income and weight, with rich people able to afford the expensive wholesome foods as well as membership in sporting clubs, while poor hard-working people may lack money for the former or time for the latter.

clouding, and incontinence. Blood tests revealed they all had gallstones, though not a one had manifested the usual pain and fever, with or without jaundice. When the gallstones were crushed or otherwise removed, the patients were able to arise and take care of themselves again. This, in itself, elevated their morale, so that a wholesome cycle was given further impetus.

To help with diagnosis of the elderly infirm, geriatric evaluation units, modeled on the successful ones in Britain, have been started in several American hospitals. One of the first was at the Veterans Administration Medical Center in Sepulveda, California. One hundred twenty-three elderly hospital patients spent time having their respective interacting ailments spotted and treated, with recommendations given for managing these on the outside. During the following year, this group turned out to have a death rate only *half* that of other elderly people, and their need for nursing-home or hospital care was *less than half* that of others. Eighty-seven percent of them, moreover, could live at home or in a housing complex for the elderly. Their lives, though perhaps not exciting, appeared to them as very much worth living.

JUNE: What was it that snapped Mary Ellen out of her doldrums and made her feel that life was worth living?

NORMAN: You can't be sure. It could have been the priest, or the doctor, or Jason's inadvertent shock treatment, or, more likely, all of them synergistically stimulating her IC.

JUNE: Is the IC essential to getting someone out of a vicious cycle?

NORMAN: Not always. Sometimes a random change in one dimension will do the trick. What never ceases to amaze me is how a minor random event, like sitting next to a child with German measles, can radically change someone's whole life, while a major event, like being in a prolonged war, doesn't appear to change some people at all.

JUNE: Yet everyone has some breaking point?

NORMAN: Oh, sure. For quite a while they can be bolstered by their significant other or by feeling themselves an integral part of a group. But if they're tortured mentally or physically for too long, they'll get sick or go crazy—or die. Going crazy, after all, isn't the worst way to block out a reality that is intolerable for that person at that time.

JUNE: What about people who don't have *enough* stress in their life, who are chronically underwhelmed?

NORMAN: That can be a real problem. Our adaptive capacities, like our muscles, need exercise. In experiments, when animals are raised in an artificially germ-free environment, some of their organs don't develop naturally. In humans who are experimentally subjected to sensory deprivation, some of their thought processes don't operate naturally. But individual humans vary so much that it's hard to predict who is going to react to what, and when.

JUNE: Don't health statistics help in predicting?

NORMAN: Only to a limited extent. What statistics show is probabilities, the way some item is distributed on a curve. But any individual at any given stage of life, or time in history, may escape the expectable cluster. The worst luck in Mary Ellen's case was the timing. A few months later or earlier than that critical period, the fetus would not have been so vulnerable.

JUNE: Yet you want our gentle reader to keep up to date about health statistics?

NORMAN: Just so he doesn't become their prisoner.

JUNE: How does that work?

NORMAN: Sometimes people take health warnings too literally. Say you're living a sedentary life and eating a lot of animal fat; you ought to know that you're increasing your chance of developing heart problems or cancer someday. But if you're an Eskimo in the winter and you let those statistics frighten you out of your share of whale blubber, you won't make it to spring.

JUNE: So in tailoring our actions to the health statistics, we need to look at the whole combo?

NORMAN: Yes. And "combo" means the IC's checking the interplay of your four dimensions.

JUNE: What about the doctor's role?

NORMAN: Doctors need to keep themselves informed about general health statistics but they also need to remain sensitive to each patient's tendency to buck some particular statistic. For example, there are patients who paradoxically react to a stimulant as if it were a tranquilizer.

JUNE: I suppose if you get too many exceptions to a rule, you have to change the rule?

NORMAN: Either that or look further for the operation of apparent randomness. Things happen that even the best scientists are surprised at.

JUNE: And the best doctors can't explain?

NORMAN: That's one reason patients should apply their scepticism whenever, like Mary Ellen, they assume too much guilt for whatever
illness or accident has occurred in their life or the life of
someone they are responsible for.

IX
Less Guilt—More Responsibility
Final Report on Sanford

"Complete freedom from disease and struggle is almost totally incompatible with the living process."
—René Dubos

Sanford, the salesman, lost forty pounds and was jogging daily when his fiancée, Esmé, asked whether she could accompany him to the psychiatrist.

"Hell no! I don't want you seeing me with my defenses down." Before she could answer, he laughed nervously. "Actually, that isn't what bothers me; I just don't think it would do any good."

"But that's what love is about, letting the other guy really know you."

"Not when what's there is so depressing."

"Depressing for whom?"

"Both of us."

"Look, Sanford, you let me handle my side of it, okay?"

"I don't see why you even want to come."

"So I can be more helpful."

"Esmé, that isn't how it works. If you come, you'll find out about you."

"So? I'll take the chance."

"Well, I'll mention it to the doc. But he probably won't want you there either."

The doctor said it would be fine if Sanford wanted Esmé to attend a few individual sessions with him. Following that, the doctor put her in a group, but not the same one as Sanford.

Within his own group, Sanford swung between worshipful agreement with the doctor and combative disagreement. In time, the group helped him see this seesaw as a pattern he tended to exhibit toward authority figures. It stemmed, he found, from his early feelings of mixed love and hate toward his brother Winthrop, who had either paid him no heed or deflated whatever brought Sanford to his attention. "When I told Winthrop I'd made the football team, he said, 'Isn't it lucky you have nothing but dinks in your class.' There was no way I could win his approval, or stop wanting to."

Gradually Sanford began to see that Winthrop had been made to feel that same way by their father. The admiral's standards for his oldest son were impossibly high. With Sanford's greater understanding of his brother—and their father—his fear of them diminished and in time he felt a poignant surge of warmth toward them.

Sanford suffered no chest pain for a year. He knew that in order to get married, he would need to ask for a raise. If the boss said no, Sanford would quit. His confidence in himself—and Esmé's in him—had grown to the point where he felt sure he could find another job.

The boss agreed to the raise!

Sanford was exultant when he met Esmé that evening. "We can get married whenever you're ready."

She burst into tears.

"Hey, you're not supposed to cry at *good* news."

"I'll cry at anything I feel like," she said. "That's one thing I learned in group."

"And when we have a child," he said, "I suppose it will be a crybaby?"

She began to laugh.

Within a few years of marriage, they had two daughters. Sanford had thought he wanted a son more than anything, but he was besotted over his little girls.

With a toddler and an infant, Esmé, however, was feeling deep frustration. Sanford could not understand her complaints. "My mother stayed home with us," he kept saying. "Besides, you've got everything you ever asked for."

They had some rough arguments. She accused him of male chauvinism; he started drinking and eating too much. His weight climbed. One day she conceded that, considering how rigid his father was, Sanford was really quite a nice open guy. "How about coming home for lunch a couple of days a week?" she suggested. "I could leave you a good salad, and go look for a part-time job."

At first Sanford balked. He did not want his precious babies bundled off to nursery school. But then he relented. Grateful that Esmé resisted arousing guilt in him for his occasional back-sliding into old habits of excess at table, he decided not to arouse guilt in her for her back-sliding into old patterns of craving the stimulation of a work place with men as well as women around. As their doctor had told them on their final session with him, "If you're lucky, you can have responsibility without too much guilt; what you have to watch out for is guilt without corresponding responsibility."

To take responsibility for one's own good health has two advantages. One is preventive: The individual assumes a self-conscious role in regard to his own habits. The other is curative: The patient decides which doctor to call in. Should disagreement arise between the doctor and the patient's own self-knowledge, or between this doctor and some other authority, the patient can decide which one to go along with.

The patient who takes responsibility for his health can usually do something about it. The very act of trying to cope, independent of its results, may boost the IC. The IC may then feel emboldened to make a new effort in another dimension, which, in turn, may speed the wholesome cycle. When Sanford finally brought himself to ask the boss for a raise, he was both conquering his outdated terror of authority figures and setting the scene for his future role as husband and father, one that by then he very much wanted and that further enhanced his sense of well-being.

A major disadvantage of taking responsibility for one's good health is that when some problem arises, one may blame oneself too severely. This overguilt may act like a negative placebo: I get sick; I needlessly castigate myself; I then feel so unworthy that I do not take care of myself; the next day the symptom is worse. Later, if the doctor I consult is visibly disappointed in my lack of improvement, I may spiral further downward.

Yet some illness is bound to occur, whether from piggy-back viruses or environmental chemicals or multiple health interactions too subtle to be spotted yet by science. Psychologist Claus Bahner Bahnson goes so far as to say that "no one is any more to blame for his illness than the features on his face; disease is so complex that to try to make any moralistic judgment about it is absurd."

Extreme self-blame in some instances becomes more debilitating than the illness itself. What some patients need is "permission" to stop being so hard on themselves and, instead, to enjoy their period of enforced rest. Even our common language may enhance guilt, as when the patient is asked, "What's *wrong* with you?" Perhaps because of America's pioneer background, the worthy individual is still expected to stay well enough to work, and if not, then quickly to pull himself up by his bootstraps. As Jory Graham writes, "Although we do not admit it, most of us feel that by sheer will power and faith, we can overcome a disease and not even feel its pain. We . . . have always believed in self-reliance, sure that with gumption and will power we could overcome any obstacle. . . . The problem with this philosophy is that when pitted against a disease, it flounders."*

The patient incapacitated in bed, the soldier confined in a prison camp, the rape victim obsessed with nightmarish recall, may all suffer from an injured IC. Having found their previous strength and ingenuity to be of no avail, their subsequent guilt and self-hatred may interfere with the success of their coping mechanisms. Stan Sommers, whose weight had dropped from 175 to 90 pounds after capture by the Japanese during World War II, later said that worse than all the malnutrition, manhandling, and tropical diseases was the sense of losing, in effect, a major component of his IC: "Once you're dependent on your captors for food, medicine, recreation, communication, every daily thing of life, you lose . . . your self-esteem."†

Some people in this situation responded with IC collapse: They gave up. E. Kincaid, author of *In Every War But One*, describes how some soldiers captured by the North Koreans first became withdrawn and sullen, apathetic and dirty, and then lay down and died. To prevent this kind of behavior from spreading, one of their leaders used "a mixture of kindly interest and anger-inducing attitudes. Victory was assumed with the first sign of a smile or evidence of pique." Another officer relied solely on anger. His aim was to make the man "so mad, by goading, prodding, or blows, that he tried to get up and beat you. If you could manage this, the man invariably got well."

These soldiers' IC "fight" reaction was probably not too different from the anger expressed by the women with advanced breast cancer who lived longer than their overly passive counterparts. Comparable to the dairy maids who had had cowpox and therefore did not contract smallpox, these women had managed to develop a valuable psychological antibody. Perhaps it derived from their self-confidence based on the knowledge that they had thus far been able to cope. Or perhaps it derived from their

*Jory Graham, *In the Company of Others* (San Diego: Harcourt Brace Jovanovich, 1978).
†Art Harris, "POWs Offer Insight Into How Hostages May Fare," *Washington Post*, 3 February 1981.

hard-won experience in how best to nurture their *body* and *mind*, seek support from *other people*, or, in some inspiriting way, improve their *environments*. Whatever their method, these women maintained their self-esteem and refused to allow overguilt to dim their eye or make them overly subservient to the authorities. By mobilizing the IC's capacity to rise above their situation at least part of the time, they metabolized the pain and did not let it degenerate into chronic suffering. As Arnold Hutschnecker, an early psychosomatic practitioner, wrote about healing, "Usually we sit and wait for the outside situation to change. But in order to get well, we ourselves must change."

Even with animals, the experience of being a responsible agent appears to have a health-improving power. Lawrence Sklar and Hymie Anison, of Carleton University in Ontario, Canada, injected three matched groups of mice with live cancer cells. While the control group was then left untouched, the other two were subjected to electric shock. One of these groups could find an escape hatch; the other could not. The trapped mice developed earlier and larger tumors, but the escaping mice developed nothing worse than the control group. Was it because they got a lift of self-esteem, a surge of brain endorphins, from their successful escapes? Certainly humans often report feeling the better for the adrenaline rush that follows their having averted or conquered a danger.

Some people who suffer from overguilt unconsciously try to load it onto other people. In transactional-analysis terms, this is the game of hot potato. (Such people may be comparable to those in a double bind who unconsciously try to put another person into one.) Sanford's father, the admiral, never stopped voicing impossible expectations for his sons.* Sanford, after recognizing this pattern and coming to relative peace with it, resolved to avoid unnecessary guilt-loading not only onto Esmé but, especially, onto his daughters. When a parent thus gives "permission" to his children to please him, he may be providing them with a major impetus toward present and future good health.

At the same time that overguilt should be avoided, so should underguilt. As a psychiatric wit put it, "We all vary between being depressive or paranoid: When depressive, we blame everything on ourselves; when paranoid, we blame it all on other people."

Somewhere in the middle lies the reasonable amount of guilt that comprises appropriate response to having made a mistake in health, as in other areas. Although guilt is an unpleasant feeling, it can be borne more readily when viewed in its wider context. "Suffering is reduced,"

---

*The admiral had been treated much the same way by *his* father. Thus are many people aptly called "the victims of victims."

says Cornell's Dr. Eric J. Cassell, "when it can be located within a coherent set of meanings."

Yet to try to absolve oneself completely from guilt when things go wrong may also have a negative effect. In a study by psychologists Helen Newman and Ellen Langer, a group of recently divorced women who felt themselves at least partially at fault (i.e., not helpless pawns) recovered their good health and spirits faster than a group who kept insisting that they had been entirely innocent.

When overguilt becomes pathological, the person himself suffers terribly, but when underguilt becomes pathological, someone else may suffer terribly. Says Willard Gaylin, M.D., "The failure to feel guilt is the basic flaw in the psychopath, or anti-social person, who is capable of committing crimes of the vilest sort without remorse or contrition," and, moreover, may even feel compelled to repeat them. *

Such people are sometimes derided as "animals," but in actuality, animals' wants are satiable, while pathological human wants, bearing, as these often do a symbolic significance, are not. Even with normal people, were anticipation of guilt not operative against violence and greed, the achievement of good health by others might be precluded.

Just as a relative few repeater criminals commit most of the major crimes, so a relatively small number of repeater patients fill most of the hospital beds. Many of them are the aged infirm who cannot help their age or, in many instances, their infirmity. But there are other patients who, with more guilt, might use their IC to break out of their long-term habits of taking four or more drinks a day, smoking a pack or more a day, forgetting to take their insulin, or persistently ignoring their doctor's advice in other ways. These people lay a heavy cost on the rest of society and might well be reminded of what the late John Knowles, M.D., called "the individual moral obligation to preserve one's own health—a public duty, if you will."

In the United States, people who fall ill may be blamed not only by society and themselves but also by their intimates, even their doctor. "*Now* what's the matter with you?" can be a guilt-loading question, and, of all people, Americans appear to be the most prone to overguilt. This tendency, in fact, came over on the *Mayflower*. To the Pilgrims, half of whom died that first winter, illness was God's punishment for individual and collective sins. Later, the New England Puritans believed that God was punishing them not only when their health failed but also when their farms or businesses did. People thought they got precisely what they deserved, either in person, or through their descendants, as the Bible

*Willard Gaylin, *Feelings* (New York: Avon Books, 1979).

had warned, "unto the third or fourth generation." Cotton Mather, apparently an early psychosomaticist, later noted that "sin brings on a sickness in the spirit [that] will naturally cause sickness of the body."

Today a health statistician looking at the mortality rate among the *Mayflower's* passengers would note many unwholesome elements. One was malnutrition—no fresh fruits or vegetables on the latter part of the journey or throughout the winter. Another was the continued, and not unjustified, anxiety about nearby hostile Indians. Still another was the bitter cold—the New England winter was harsher than any they had known. From a psychosomatic angle, it may be significant that their much-relied-on spiritual leader, William Brewster, and their much-relied-on military leader, Myles Standish, were among the few who did not catch the prevalent disease, despite their arduous nursing of those who had.

At the turn of the twentieth century, Freud, an atheist, rejected the role of God as punisher in time of illness or rewarder in time of wellness. While removing one source of guilt from patients, he ironically added another. This was the unconscious force within the individual that may contribute to illness and also to the kind of so-called accident that, until then, had been attributed to God's will or simply bad luck. Today, as a result of Freud's views, even the victim of *someone else's* accident or bad luck (in your tumble, you knock me over) may be offered criticism rather than comfort. The theory is that I may be at fault for having attracted your unconscious hostility. Apparent randomness and true accident, therefore, need to be remembered when blame for injury or illness is too blithely assumed or handed out.

It was no accident that the country most hospitable to Freud's ideas was the United States. As reflected in the Declaration of Independence, Americans have long emphasized the significance of the individual. And psychoanalysis is the most individual-centered of the healing disciplines.

In the United States, individuals in recent years have been suffering from overguilt, not only for their own ailments and accidents but also for those of their children.

This tendency accelerated after World War II, when Freud's concepts were first widely disseminated. Many self-proclaimed experts from diverse disciplines advised parents that if they would just avoid the glaring mistakes made by their Victorian predecessors, the new generation would grow up healthier and happier than human beings had ever been.

The primary step, said these experts, was for parents to offer the children "unconditional love." When many merely human women and men found this command to be impossible on a full-time basis, their self-confidence, self-image, and even IC, were eroded. They therefore began handling their children so guiltily that they lost one of the virtues of their Victorian predecessors—namely, their self-certainty.

Modern parents have also been confused about what kind of experience causes children merely to feel *frustration* and what causes them to engage in *repression*.

By the late 1970s, the most influential of the so-called experts, the venerable pediatrician Benjamin Spock, was himself suffering from severe guilt. As he said with his characteristic honesty in San Diego in 1979, "The big problem is that parents constantly worry about whether they are doing the right thing. Nowadays, there are more parents who are afraid of their children than children who are afraid of their parents. And this is the first time in the history of the human race that this has ever happened. We have psychologists, social workers, teachers—telling parents what they should and shouldn't do. And this has robbed parents of confidence in their own judgment. . . . Now I realize that the most valuable thing for me to do is help parents have confidence. Now I tell parents, 'You know more than you think you do.' "

Just as the medical sciences are moving beyond the single-cause theory of illness, the social and behavioral sciences are now moving beyond the simple blaming of parents for a child's current or later ills. The 1981 report of the Carnegie Council on Children, for example, recommends that much of the blame for children's problems be shifted from parents to the wider community. Factors such as the media have a greater impact on some aspects of child development than the few hours a week the child spends with one or both parents.*

Much of the responsibility for a child's well-being has been placed back on the individual child in order to give him the chance to develop IC strength through decision-making. A sense of control, of having one's choices matter, may counter what psychologist Martin Seligman calls "learned helplessness" in childhood. This kind of copelessness may make children more vulnerable to stress at the time, and also later. Unconsciously, they may give up in despair, he says, not because their situation is objectively hopeless but because they have learned from their own experience that they can neither fight nor flee nor successfully join with others to change their situation.

Learned helplessness, moreover, may develop when a child is overly indulged as well as when he is overly frustrated. If too many good things happened during his childhood with no IC effort on his part, the child

---

*The number of single-parent households in the United States has increased by 80 percent in the past ten years, with one family in five now having a single parent.

may not learn the skills or self-reliance necessary for later competence. Instead he may become an emotional or geographic drifter. *

On the other side of the coin, the development of such IC skills may be precisely what was forced on a group of inner-city youngsters from emotionally and financially deprived homes who rose to good health and fortune later on. Psychoanalyst Erik Erikson, Harvard professor emeritus, suggests that these youngsters may have found through their active street life with peers both the support and challenge that their parent(s) could not provide.

"Controllable stress," rather than a trauma-free childhood, is now recommended for the young. A dramatic example is the Outward Bound program. Through climbing sheer rock and surviving for days alone without rations in the woods, young people form both a new self-esteem and a realistic awareness of their limits. The importance of the latter was pointed to by Thomas J. Watson, Sr., the founder of IBM. "Failure is a teacher—a harsh one, but the best; pull your failures to pieces looking for the reasons, and then put them to work for you."

To do this presupposes a resilient IC. And IC power is also necessary to pulling one's overguilt to pieces, in order both to learn from it and to reduce it to manageable proportions. A first step may be conscious recognition: to call overguilt, like Rumpelstiltskin, by its name and thus reduce its power. A second may be to ventilate one's painful anxiety to a pastor, doctor, or friend whose judgment one respects. A third may be to program one's unconscious to go in the desired direction, and then let time, distance, and the mysterious processes of internal readjustment do their work of pain relief and self-bolstering.

In all events, parents should no longer suffer too much guilt for what went wrong while their children were growing up, and if the child refuses to accept at least some of the responsibility for whatever his current woe, they might offer the version of "tough love" called *parentectomy* (removal of parent from daily contact with the child). † Without the daily abrasiveness, scabs can form over wounds for both generations, and in time the wounds may heal.

---

*This theory is supported by child-specialist Jean Macfarlane's thirty-year study of two hundred children. The biggest surprise was the later unhappiness and immaturity of boys and girls who had grown up under seemingly optimal conditions at home and gone on to be high-school athletic stars or remarkable for their good looks and popularity. Too much success too easily earned may have prevented IC development. Or perhaps, as Ben Franklin noted, "Those things that hurt, instruct."

†The child might live with some other relative for a while, or, if on drugs, then in a rehabilitation center. Summer camp also offers a mutually profitable vacation for both generations.

It is typical for a child to visualize a parent in terms of a few freeze-frames—as when a movie stops and holds a scene for longer than the usual interval. But such freeze-frames are often less characteristic of the specific parent than of the archetype he has come to represent. The child, for example, may picture the parent of the same sex with fist upraised. Yet when, through the child's maturing—or perhaps therapy—the inner film gets moving again, the fist dissolves into a hand that, in mistaken playfulness, had been hiding a piece of candy. As a modern observer of intergenerational tension has stated, "It's never too late to have had a happy childhood."

For child as well as parent, guilt for real wrongdoing may be easier to deal with than guilt for imaginary wrongdoing. If a child is miserable because his parents are disappointed in his performance, there are several steps available. One is for him to get to work and improve it. Another is for the parents to become more realistic in their expectations. A third is for the child to mobilize his IC, realizing that he can only do his best, and is not to blame if the result does not happen to suit them. (The last is what Sanford did.) But if the child's guilt is imaginary in nature, then whatever praise the parents offer may be misinterpreted by him ("You're just soft-soaping me because you have no faith that I could do better"), and his guilt may continue, perhaps long after they have died.

In addition to having one's guilt be realistic, it should be aroused primarily by one's acts that are deliberate, not unintentional. One of the most painful scenes in all literature is when Oedipus puts out his eyes because of what he had unwittingly done to his father and mother. His self-blinding, moreover, not only failed to help them but added a further burden to his long-suffering daughters, who, thereafter, had to lead him around by the hand.

What Oedipus was suffering was remorse, which has been defined as regret without hope, or despair. While regret can be as profound as remorse, it includes the possibility of improvement. Perhaps one can make amends, or so change oneself that the hurtful act will never be repeated, or one may be forgiven.

Forgiveness, the great absolver of overguilt, has been paid more heed by the religions than by the sciences or philosophies. In Judaism and Christianity, the importance of forgiveness by God and human beings is central. And, in effect, the message is the same: *Forgiveness does not need first to be deserved.* It can come as a "gift," without strings, and when accepted, it may provide a "new life" in which helplessness is dissolved and hopelessness revised.

Sometimes recovery from illness presupposes a form of forgiveness. As Miriam Siegler and Humphrey Osmond write about patienthood, "The central issue in convalescence is forgiveness. . . . Recovery depends on accepting the sick role, which means you do not blame yourself or others for your illness. If you are still blaming yourself . . . you will tend to push yourself beyond what you can do at your stage of recovery and . . . suffer a relapse. If you blame others, you will be tempted to do too little."*

Some people have actually been brought back from the brink of death by an expression of forgiveness. Such forgiveness may come from an individual once harmed by the patient or, as in the Catholic "ceremony for the sick" (formerly "extreme unction"), from a general assurance of God's mercy.

Forgiveness, moreover, is one of the most effective ways to break into a vicious cycle between two people who keep bringing out the worst in each other. Sometimes forgiving is linked with forgetting; sometimes it is defined as grace or *agape*, the kind of love that is "heedless of self." Shakespeare delegated to one of his most vibrant and pragmatic characters, a lawyer, the job of defining it. Says Portia in *The Merchant of Venice*:

> The quality of mercy is not strain'd
> It droppeth as the gentle rain from heaven
> Upon the place beneath: it is twice bless't;
> It blesseth him that gives and him that takes.

"Twice bless't" is an elegant version of "It takes two to tango." Just as illness needs a noxious agent plus a vulnerable host, so forgiveness needs a willing donor and a willing receiver, a person who will drop his previous unproductive behavior in order to make the changes entailed by his acceptance of the forgiveness. Sometimes forgiver and forgivee are the same person.

The openness of forgiveness contrasts with the closedness of the unconscious defenses. These raise barriers in order to protect the tender core of the self, while to accept forgiveness involves the risk of lowering one's barriers. On the other hand, if forgiveness is offered prematurely or in the form of a blank check, its healing power may be dissipated. For people to receive forgiveness in fruitful fashion, they need first to have become aware of why it is needed. Yet this kind of awareness can temporarily shatter the person to the very marrow of his IC.

In fact, if the ship of self is not well balanced, the person may be

---

*Miriam Siegler and Humphrey Osmond, *How to Cope With Illness: Dealing With Your Doctor, Your Relatives, and Yourself When You Are Ill* (New York: Macmillan, 1981).

terrified of sinking if faced with a fundamental need for self-blame or change. Instead, like Dorothy, such a person may unconsciously deny the need and try, by projection or displacement, to keep foisting it off onto someone else.

On the other hand, if the ship of self is relatively well balanced, the IC can afford to take aboard the load of having erred. In the short run, people who risk believing they were mistaken feel an upsurge of painful anxiety and may even develop a symptom of some sort. But in the long run, the effect of confronting one's need for forgiveness may result in a blessed relief, a lightening of an unconscious burden that the person had not recognized as such, and a strengthening of the IC for the future.

Sometimes, as when Peter arrived at the bedside of his former wife, Martha, who was dying of pneumonia, the attempt to be reconciled comes so late that the person to whom one wanted to make amends is beyond reach. Mary Ellen, on the other hand, after her engagement to Jason, was able to forgive her mother for the harshness shown while Mary Ellen was growing up.

Although the person from whom one wants forgiveness may be dying, or even dead, the chain of healing is not necessarily broken. For with regret, which includes hope, one can make restitution, if not to the original person, then to someone else. Older individuals, for example, may be especially generous to a young person, in order indirectly to repay someone long dead for major kindness shown when they were too callow to express appreciation for it. Thus a wholesome interpersonal cycle, as well as the vicious variety, can continue "unto the third or fourth generation."

People who cannot accept forgiveness are likely also to be those who cannot offer it. They burnish their grudges rather than relinquishing them. Yet the grudge may end up as more of a burden to them than to the person who elicited it. From the hospital, Zelda Fitzgerald wrote, "I am physically and mentally ravaged by resentment." Such people, in psychiatrist Edmund Bergler's phrase, are "the injustice collectors."

Yet if the aggrieved party can shift from subjective to objective gear, he might spot an explanation for the original cause of the grievance. From that explanation might arise the kind of understanding that resembles forgiveness (like Sanford's spotting the strains put on his brother by their father). Such understanding may also interrupt a long-term vicious cycle in the culprit, of bad behavior leading to overguilt and self-hatred, leading to worse behavior and further guilt.

Said Alexander Pope, "To err is human; to forgive, divine." And similarly divine, at times, is to forget. People often say, "Oh, forget it" or "Never mind" or "You can't win 'em all" or "That's life." Thus do they convey the welcome news that they are refraining from investing emotional energy in their grievance.

While some people with a weakened IC may overapologize, others cannot gird themselves to say things like "I goofed" or "My mistake" or "I didn't mean it" or "Please forgive me." Said a middle-aged man who finally learned the relief that may stem from such honest admission, "It took me more than forty years to realize that I didn't have to be perfect in order to be loved."

NORMAN: Okay, June, this time I'm going to start the questions. How come you and Jonathan get along so well with your kids?

JUNE: Because they're old enough to be forgiving. Also, we all lucked out in regard to their genes. When I think of some that they might have inherited!

NORMAN: You know you're being fashionable by stressing genetics?

JUNE: Really?

NORMAN: Blaming everything on your physical genes—and the particular neurotransmitter pattern based on them—has taken the place of blaming everything on your childhood traumas.

JUNE: But how can you do anything about your genes? At least with your parents' mistakes, you can try to understand what made them act that way.

NORMAN: Not all genes are beyond modification. Only the central ones. What we mostly inherit are predispositions.

JUNE: Like what?

NORMAN: Well, let's say there's a genetic factor in alcoholism. Sanford's father, the old admiral, is a heavy drinker. But that doesn't mean that Sanford has to do the same. He can avoid it by *not* drinking. In other words, these genetic factors don't work in any exact, one-to-one way.

JUNE: So it's the old business of the combo?

NORMAN: Absolutely. The IC! There's the predisposition, on the one hand, and what the person decides to do about it on the other. Sanford has deliberately made himself different from his father.

JUNE: Don't lots of people bend over backward to be different from their parent of the same sex?

NORMAN: They do. Look at who Sanford married. His mother was mousy, so he marries Esmé, who is strong and outspoken. Yet one of his and Esmé's daughters may turn out to be just like her mousy grandmother.

JUNE: Would that be the genes?

NORMAN: It might. Or it might be the child's unconsciously trying to establish herself as different from *her* mother. A lot of take-charge women, like Esmé, find it hard to drop back to the slower rhythms of little kids.

JUNE: There's a book out with a swell title: *How to Talk So Kids Will Listen, and Listen So Kids Will Talk*. In that sense, today's parents are a big improvement over the past. Also, they no longer openly play favorites.

NORMAN: Yet unwittingly, a parent may reward the child who is most like himself. I enjoy the way your kids are so different from you and Jonathan—and from each other.

JUNE: It makes life interesting. Who needs a lot of clones?

NORMAN: Some parents seem to. They grow anxious—or critical—when their child chooses a life-style different from their own. Unless the child imitates them, they fear they must have been wrong. There seems to be some free-floating guilt between parents and children—like the free-floating anxiety that Freud spotted.

JUNE: Is that because family members are too judgmental about each other?

NORMAN: There's a time for judging—and for suspending judgment. A key time for suspending it is when someone gets sick. Perhaps it was the fault of the patient's genes; perhaps it was the fault of his behavior; but the main thing is not to make him feel too guilty. Just because humans are capable of imagining perfection doesn't mean that we're capable of achieving it. And the irony is that if people would strain less for perfect health— or perfect parenthood—they might feel—and act—a whole lot better.

JUNE: And their doctor would be more pleased with them?

NORMAN: Right! Doctors wouldn't be able to maintain their households if *none* of their patients got sick; but they wouldn't be able to maintain their sanity if *all* their patients got sick at the same time.

X

The Activated Patient and the Liberated Doctor

Final Report on Dorothy

> *"Programming people to do much more about their own health would be a lot more economical and effective than producing more doctors. Patients are an immense, untapped health manpower resource."*
> —Professor Eli Ginzberg, Columbia University

> *"The doctor of the future will give no medicine but will interest his patients in the care of the human frame, in diet, and in cause and prevention of disease."*
> —Thomas A. Edison

The psychiatrist who tried to help Dorothy with her intensifying problems with her husband at home and with her fellow nurses at work heard nothing for several years after her abrupt departure. Then one day the psychiatrist received a call from an internist on the staff of a nearby general hospital. Dorothy had been admitted because of bleeding ulcers. The psychiatrist was frank with the internist about Dorothy's unconscious tendency to switch from physical to mental symptoms and back again, meanwhile blaming everyone except herself for her ailment.

A few months later the internist reported back. Dorothy's ulcers had improved and she was discharged, but now she was threatening to sue the hospital because of her claim that one of their medications had given her migraine.

More than a year later, the psychiatrist received a call from a nearby psychiatric hospital. Dorothy had been brought in suffering from "paranoid ideation." Her father, she insisted, had been phoning the nurses she worked with, and now the ones who took care of her, to laugh about her behind her back. She was begging to see her old psychiatrist.

One day, after visiting another hospital patient, the doctor stopped by. Dorothy was a mountain of flaccid flesh. "I've tried so hard to lose weight," she told the doctor. "I went to a fat farm and paid a thousand dollars, but all I lost was seven pounds. They cheated me."

"When did the extra weight start?"

"After my mother died. I had worked night and day to get her and my father together. I'll never forgive her for turning her back on him."

"And he?"

Her eyes narrowed. "He's crazy. After Mother died, I helped him move to a new apartment. But he never appreciated the curtains I made. And he began phoning the nurses I worked with . . ."

The psychiatrist talked with Dorothy's doctor and the hospital social worker. They agreed on prescribing a new combination of psychoactive drugs and an exercise class for Dorothy. As Dorothy's contact with reality increased, she became less obsessed with food. She began losing weight and feeling better and losing more weight.

The social worker visited Peter. She explained that Dorothy had always loved her father and needed occasional signs of love from him. If Peter could offer approval now and then instead of always criticizing—or, even better, if he could cease judging her as if she were an errant child and simply enjoy her adult company—she might improve sufficiently to be released from the hospital. Peter nodded, and in time Dorothy was released, thus reducing both her unhappiness and the sizable health bill that was being paid in part by her insurance company and in part, indirectly, by her fellow taxpayers.

Health care has become the third largest industry in the U.S. (the other two being construction and agriculture). In 1983 the national medical bill was $355.4 billion, 10.8 percent of the gross national product, an average of $1,459 per person.

Did people get their money's worth?

Some of them, some of the time, certainly did, especially those who learned enough about their own health to aid their doctor in his attempts to aid them.

During previous centuries, it made little difference whether patients had an inkling of what their doctor was trying to do. For most of what he did was to administer emetics (to cause vomiting), purges (to cause diarrhea), or leeches (to drain the body of unwanted blood), mostly to no avail, and sometimes to the detriment of the patient's health. The death of George Washington, for example, was probably hastened by his conscientious doctors, who, because of his badly inflamed throat, bled him and thus added to his debilitation.

On the other hand, doctors in those days—like Victorian parents—had the self-confidence that stemmed from awareness that they knew all there was to know about the subject. Emanating this confidence often added to the placebo effect of their advice.

Today, in contrast, doctors are repeatedly reminded of how little they know, even about their specialty, let alone its relationship to the many other specialties. And being forced to make life-or-death decisions on the basis of inadequate, even contradictory, information is extremely stressful. Sometimes doctors deny their ignorance and are unpleasantly surprised when patients raise questions about diagnosis or treatment. In the United States and Britain, three times as many doctors commit suicide or become alcoholics as the rest of the population. Among women doctors, the death rate is three times greater than among men doctors.*

Beginning with premed courses and continuing through the specialty boards, the doctor must master a huge amount of factual information. Repeatedly, examinations based on this knowledge will determine his professional future. Internship and residency entail severe overwork and lack of sleep, interrupted home life and alarming crises with patients. It is almost as if these healthy young men and women were being deliberately reduced in well-being so that they could develop understanding for the kind of fatigue, debilitation, and distortion of judgment that many patients suffer.

What is often omitted, both in selection of medical students and in their training, is the encouragement of compassion rather than dispassion. What is needed is more encouragement of those human perceptions that enable doctors to treat each patient as a singular individual, not merely a fleshly envelope in which symptoms are being delivered for their expert appraisal. Insufficiently heeded by many doctors is the early-twentieth-century advice of Dr. Francis Weld Peabody, a professor of internal medicine at Harvard, that "the secret of the care of the patient is caring for the patient."

In 1984, the medical community was jolted when Harvard's president, Derek Bok, criticized American medical schools in general—and Har-

*Figures used by neurologist Sir John Walton in a speech before the British Medical Association on October 21, 1981.

vard's in particular—for their continued neglect of those arts called *humane.*

The usual hospital setup remains almost military: a "war" against disease, involving a rigid hierarchy of officers (doctors), noncoms (nurses), and soldiers (health aides and technicians). Frequently, information is shared from above, like wartime secrets, only on a need-to-know basis. Many senior doctors do not take time to fill in the interns; many interns do not take time to fill in the nurses; many nurses do not take time to fill in the health aides, and many patients are left puzzled and unnecessarily frightened.

Says medical anthropologist John-Henry Pfifferling, "Most of the orderlies and technicians have no idea why they do what they do. There's no sense of teamwork. Everyone's left out except the doctors, which means that they're not only terribly overburdened, but also resented by their co-workers. . . . Docs are trained to believe that they must always appear all-knowing. They have no preparation for failure. They're highly competitive and tend not to support their colleagues when they're having a hard time. They're trained to focus on problems, not strengths; facts, not feelings."*

With an average of three hundred thousand Americans being hospitalized each year because of adverse reactions to drugs prescribed by doctors, some drastic change in health care is long overdue. Once in the hospital, moreover, 10 percent of patients develop infections, some of these from microbes that have become drug-resistant because antibiotics had been inappropriately prescribed.

By and large, doctors and patients each divide into two groups. There are the authoritarian doctors and the liberated ones. There are the acquiescent patients and the activated ones. When an authoritarian doctor and an acquiescent patient get together, all may be well. Similarly, when a liberated doctor and an activated patient get together, all may be well. But when an authoritarian doctor is faced with an activated patient—or a liberated doctor with an acquiescent patient—serious effort to avoid misunderstanding may be needed on both sides.

One liberated doctor, for example, had a patient so acquiescent that she took everything he said quite literally. "You've been overworking," he said. "Go home, go to bed, act as if you had a bad cold, and call me after three days."

Three days later, to the minute, she phoned. "I did what you said and acted as if I had a cold. But I just wasn't able to cough."

*Tom Ferguson, M.D., "The Wounded Healers, A Conversation with John-Henry Pfifferling," *Medical Self Care*, Fall 1980.

"That isn't quite what I meant," he answered. "But did the bed rest make you feel any better?"

"No, I don't think so," she said in a dispirited voice.

More successful was an authoritarian psychiatrist with an activated patient who had been suffering from feelings of unworthiness. At work she was supposed to phone a major expert in her field to get his opinion on a problem. But she felt too anxious to do so. Her boss pressed her, which increased her anxiety. The longer she delayed, the less worthy she felt.

Her doctor offered her considerable emotional support and, as she was leaving, said, "Make the call; don't be afraid."

The next day she did it. She said she could hear in her head the doctor's voice saying, "Go on, don't be afraid," even as she was dialing. Having successfully completed the call, she phoned the doctor. "It seems so obvious," she said. "All I had to do was just *do* it."

He told her how pleased he was that it had worked out. But even if it had not, he said, she would have learned something. She might have learned that failure is not the worst thing in the world, or that one's anxiety about an event is often worse than the event. Also, having tried it once, she would probably find it easier to do the next time. In this instance, his no-nonsense command had been more effective than a lot of psychiatric explanation.

A less fortunate example was reported by an activated mother in relation to her sons' authoritarian pediatrician: "Our youngest child . . . is an asthmatic. He had recently . . . been put on slo-phyllin [a bronchodilator]. . . . While grateful to the [drug], I had, on occasion, asked our pediatrician about its side-effects. I had also noticed the orange label on the hydrocandalupent-dimentane medication and the statement that it was a 'controlled substance.' I called our pediatrician . . . to ask whether our son's medication had narcotics in it. He said he did not know and recommended I call my pharmacist."*

Later she called the pediatrician to ask his opinion of mega-doses of vitamins. The doctor's response, she said, "was quite emotional. 'Those people who recommend such doses,' he yelled, 'they are a bunch of quacks just interested in your money!' " He then sent her a certified letter dismissing her children as his patients. Her boys, she reported, were furious with her. She explained that, in their best interest, a doctor was needed who would welcome, rather than feel threatened by, their mother's informed questions.

A happy example of an acquiescent patient with an authoritarian doctor

*Evelyn Jackson, "Coping: The 'Why' Syndrome," *Washington Post*, 17 September 1980.

was Peter when first brought to the hospital in a state of total disorientation. He was so relieved to have someone doing something for him that he followed all the doctor's instructions and mended with a speed that surprised everyone.

When patient and doctor are well suited, an important factor in their success may be the meshing of their expectations for treatment. If the doctor is confident that the patient will recover, the patient's IC may be stimulated into making an extra effort. By doing well, he then proves the doctor correct, which makes for a wholesome cycle. But if the doctor has no hope, the patient may also pick up on this and fade all the faster. In *The Broken Heart*, Doctor James J. Lynch compares the doctor's bedside manner to the observer in Heisenberg's principle of indeterminacy: Just as the physicist cannot observe an electron without changing it, so the physician cannot react to his patient without changing him.

What is true of physicians appears to be equally true of nurses and other hospital staff. In an experiment at the University of Denver Medical Center, two groups of coronary patients were matched for age, sex, and degree of impairment. One group had a liaison psychiatrist assigned to work both with patients and staff members; the other did not. Over time, the first group had a one-third lower mortality rate than the second group. Then, when the liaison psychiatrist was reassigned, the first group's rate climbed up to match the second group's.*

So great an effect can the doctor's expectations have that some terminal patients have hung onto life well beyond the point of its being anything but agony to them and everyone else, because they did not want to disappoint their doctor. Dr. David Murray of the Oxford Hospice in England explicitly gives such patients permission to let go—and gratefully they do so. He, among other hospice doctors, agrees with the dictum of the late Dr. Edward Trudeau, founder of the Saranac, N.Y., Hospital: "Sometimes cure, often help, and always console."

Other times it is the *patient's* own hope that energizes the *doctor*. In *A World to Care For*, Howard A. Rusk, M.D., recalls the early days of the New York University rehabilitation center that now bears his name: "We were . . . learning that you don't tell handicapped people what they can't do, because you're never sure they aren't able to do it until you see them try."

As important as the doctor's expectations for the patient are the patient's expectations for himself. Sometimes the unconscious defense, denial, encourages patients to perform beyond statistical probability. For ex-

*Reported to Dr. Tamarkin on the phone by Dr. Stephen Dubovsky, chief of liaison psychiatry, University of Denver Medical Center, October 1984.

ample, most women with only one lung or one kidney or severe diabetes
are advised by doctors not to try to bear a child. But some women have
refused to believe that the discouraging numbers would apply to *them*.
Instead, they have become pregnant and successfully given birth.

In certain patients, the sense of control involved in a bit of defiance
toward their doctor boosts their IC. Some first-time heart-disease sufferers,
for example, indulged themselves in food treats not included in their
restricted diet. Their rate of recovery was better than that of comparable
patients who were so stunned by the seriousness of their condition that
they meticulously followed the doctor's every instruction. *

A larger example of defiance is offered by the town of Framingham,
Massachusetts. While it is the site of the nation's longest study of heart
disease (source of the original warnings against ingesting too much cholesterol), Framingham also supports just as many fast-food outlets as any
other small town. Of course, this fact does not negate the worth of health
warnings in general, since so many individuals in Framingham and
elsewhere have given up smoking. Perhaps what it indicates is simply
that now and then the IC needs to assert itself as unique by a relatively
innocent thumbing of the nose at statistics and scientists.

Today, even the most acquiescent patient who goes to the most authoritarian doctor needs to take more health responsibility than he might
have in the past. For the patient's self-observations (ideally kept as a daily
log) are useful to the doctor, both for his diagnosis and for monitoring
of today's typically many-faceted treatment. The patient's reported sensations are often the trip-wire that alerts the doctor to ask questions about
drugs or vitamins or nutrients that the patient is taking.

In order to facilitate the patient's willingness to communicate, three
words are worth dropping from the medical lexicon. One is *uncomfortable*
as a euphemism for "painful." Few things are more disconcerting than
to have spent a sleepless night in agony only to hear the nurse report in
the morning that the patient had been "uncomfortable." Another word
is *complaint*, with its implication of whininess; instead, "symptom," "clue,"
"discomfort," or "pain" could be used. In return, the patient might be
careful to distinguish between "pain" and mere "discomfort," even though
the latter, when chronic or combined with other forms of (di)stress, may
be harder on the IC than isolated pain that is short-lived.

Finally, there is the adjective *unremarkable* as applied to "recovery."
To the patient, no recovery is unremarkable ("Happiness," said tough
old newsman Walter Duranty, "is relief from pain.") Few experiences
are more poignant and miraculous than the springlike sensations of re-

*Clinical Psychiatry News, April 1981.

turning good health. Some doctors at such times, however, make the patient feel boring, as if wasting valuable professional time, and are impatient with mundane but personally important questions such as when the patient should return to work or pre-ailment diet or sexual activity.

From their side, patients might exercise restraint in asking their doctor's advice on extraneous matters. Said an exhausted internist, "At the end of the day, I feel like the receiving end of Dial-A-Friend." And one pediatrician bewailed the case of a couple who made an appointment to ask him whether they should send their child to Sunday School.

Sometimes more useful to the patient tha the doctor is the nurse, and making friends with the nurse, whether in office or hospital, is a valuable form of health insurance. In fact, a quiet revolution is taking place in the relationship between patients and nurses, as well as between nurses and doctors. Nurses are not only better trained than ever before but also have higher expectations for what their job should entail. Being skilled in health-nursing as well as sick-nursing, they are often the patient's best source of practical information about how to get well and stay well. And patients often find them easier to be frank with than the doctor.

The best nurses, like the best doctors, are sometimes unsung heroes in the tender, loving care they provide for patients with diseases, like AIDS, that are simultaneously contagious and potentially lethal.

As for the nurse-doctor relationship, this is no longer based on what used to be called the "benevolent conspiracy," namely, keeping the patient in the dark. Nurses tend to believe, more than do traditional doctors, that the patient does better if given facts, both about himself and about the relevant elements of curative and preventive medicine. On the other hand, nurses, like doctors, need to be careful *not* to overload with detailed information the patient who is either not interested or so anxious that he is likely to misinterpret what is said. * By and large, in one way or another, patients manage to make known how much they really want to be told.

Especially useful to the convalescent patient are relatives or friends with previous experience of managing illness. They are the ones likely to give good common-sense advice: "You can't hurry Mother Nature" or "This kind of thing takes a lot out of you" or "Convalescence is one step backward for each two steps forward."

This common-sense person may be the patient's significant other, and both doctor and nurse need to offer support to the SO. Especially when an illness drags on and on, the role of well spouse or well parents or well

---

*New forms of competitiveness have also arisen between some doctors and some of the new supertrained nurses, with the result that they do not coordinate their advice, and the patient is left confused about how to act.

offspring may be riddled with conflict between the needs of the patient and the needs of self; nor may the guilt of such conflict disappear after the death of the patient. Colin Murray Parkes, M.D., author of *On Bereavement*, suggests that writers of condolence letters include a kind word about the recipient as well as the deceased, for the bereaved person, like Jason, may be suffering not only from grief but also from a worn-down IC. As Dr. Parkes puts it, "The usual capacity for self-love becomes impaired."

Dr. Elisabeth Kubler Ross, the Swiss thanatologist (expert on death and dying), suggests that bereaved people go through many, if not all, of the five stages she identifies as experienced by the dying themselves— namely, denial, anger, bargaining, depression, and, finally, acceptance.

Physical as well as emotional symptoms often arise in the SO following the loved one's death. In a 1980 study of recent widowers, Dr. Marvin Stein, chairman of the psychiatry department at New York's Mount Sinai Medical Center, reported on "the marked changes in their lymph cells which help guard against disease." With the person's immune system thus undermined, all kinds of diseases may attack and further weaken the person's resistance. Alert doctors—and family members and friends— pay special attention to the bereaved person for at least six months.

Some bereaved people slump into apathy and deep depression. Others become temporarily hectic, as if, through constant activity, they could hold their grief at bay. Yet after the widow(er) has had time and incentive to work though the grief, a new plateau of good health and spirits may be achieved.

On the other hand, there are some people who blossom at the time of the serious illness, even death, of their spouse. Peter, for example, had responded to his wife Martha's post-partum depression (following the birth of Dorothy) by getting himself assigned to the night shift and taking care of the baby by day. He enjoyed the responsibility and the baby's crow of joy at the sight of him. When Martha was finally released from the hospital, Peter sagged in all dimensions, and refused to do anything further of a personal nature for the child.

Other people sicken, apparently, because of a profound loss suffered by someone else. Kenneth Pelletier, clinical psychologist at The University of California Medical School in San Francisco, reports a study of wives who fell ill when their husband lost his job. In some women, the cholesterol level went up; in others, respiratory symptoms developed. From a statistical point of view, to have one's spouse in good working order is a useful form of health insurance.

Yet if one lives long enough, grievous losses to self or family members are bound to occur. And it is at such times that physical or emotional ailments are most likely to surface. Bereavement, in fact, heads the Social Readjustment Rating Scale devised at the Naval Health Research Center in San Diego by Drs. Richard H. Rahe and Thomas H. Holmes. In this scale (see Appendix B), what they termed Life Change Units (LCU's) are listed in the order of frequency with which they were reported by a large group of hospital patients as having taken place during the year that preceded their illness.

The events are by no means only unhappy ones. High on the list of stressful occasions is a couple's reconciliation after a separation. Midway down the list are marriage and the arrival of a new family member. Others are new job, new home, new success. A sexual problem is at about the same stress level as pregnancy. More than half of the events concern relationships with other people, though some, such as moving, also involve environments. Yet moving, which for some people is "the only thing that gets *harder* with practice," is a welcome challenge for others: "I'm growing restless," said a diplomat's wife after two years in the same post. "I hope we get a new assignment soon."

Differences appear between individuals—and between the same individual and himself at different ages—in regard to the effects of a specific LCU. Differences also appear between individuals' tolerances for a high total of LCU's at different times. Dr. Rahe notes that although some sicken, "There are far more who do not go on to report illness than those who do."

When stress buildup becomes too much for a person, he might well ask himself if his behavior is suitable to his age-group. Some people at forty continue to run as hard as at fourteen; some at fourteen try alone to resolve conflicts that a person of forty would refer to a professional. What is relaxing at one stage may become stressful at another. The parental cuddling needed by the small child may be loathed by the adolescent, or the rock music loved by the adolescent may be anathema to the adult. If a couple quarrels, their small child may panic; their adolescent may blame himself; their contemporary may worry about his own marriage; and their elderly friend may be philosophical, for, from the perspective of experience, the old one may know that between people who love, some anger is inevitable.

The older person may also have learned, probably the hard way, the lesson of "enoughness." This was described by psychoanalyst Lawrence Kubie as one of the touchstones of mental health: "the freedom to cease when sated." Even when not entirely sated, people may need their IC at times to prevent them from straining for still more or better. A current definition of mental health is "the ability to live fully in the present," in effect, neither haunted by one's own or other people's mistakes in the past, nor by insatiability in the present, nor by perfectionist expectations for the future.*

Enoughness is important also in regard to medical treatment. If a familiar drug is working well, why experiment with the newest one? If a simple diagnosis makes sense, why try to rule out every conceivable disease that, under the most unusual circumstances, might be causing the same symptoms? Sometimes doctors, gun-shy about being sued, practice defensive medicine. Fearing accusations of malpractice for doing too little, they do too much, in terms of both the patient's suffering and his impoverishment.† The patient or his SO may need to say no to some tests, especially those of the invasive variety. The patient or his SO may also need to say no to hospitalization, especially for the elderly infirm.

Until around 1950, the majority of the elderly died at home, surrounded by beloved people and objects. But today 80 percent die in medical institutions, not only with strangers and sterile furnishings around them but also, often, with hated tubes going into them. Unfortunately, neither nursing-home nor home care is generally covered by private insurance or Medicare. Yet the hospital is often the worst place to do one's dying, because its red tape and constant chaperonage by doctors and nurses prevent the disconnecting of invasive tubes even when the aged, anguished, and moribund patient had begged for this form of release.

"Old age," as a ninety-year-old Vassar graduate wrote to her alumnae magazine, "is not for sissies." Yet the deprivations of old age may provide the incentive to develop new IC skills. Said author and critic Malcolm Cowley on his eightieth birthday, "The people I envy are those who accept old age as a series of challenges. For them each new infirmity is an enemy to be outwitted, an obstacle to be overcome by force of will, and they enjoy each little victory over themselves."

Though youth is often touted as "the best years of your life," many an elder would refuse to relinquish his hard-won IC strength in order to return to young people's typical insecurities. Later in life, because the four dimensions tend to be no longer so imperious in their demands, the person may enjoy a greater sense of IC control. This control, besides

---

*Even that insatiable seeker of sensation, Walt Whitman, finally wrote:

"I have perceived that to be with those I like is enough,
To stop in company with the rest at evening is enough."

Implied by him is not only relationship with other people, but also the evening meal (body), stimulating conversation (mind), and a pleasant ambience (environments).

†In 1983 sixteen malpractice suits were filed for every 100 doctors, and total awards to suing patients came to two billion dollars.

being intrinsically pleasant, may be a useful ingredient in a harmonious patient-doctor relationship.

For patients with less self-knowledge and experience, this relationship often reactivates unconscious childish attachments to authority figures that interfere with optimal treatment. The patient may become overly anxious to please or overly rebellious, confusingly flirtatious or quick to take offense. But whatever his attitude, it is likely *not* to be grounded in the here-and-now, as Dorothy's attitude toward her various doctors never was.

On the doctor's side, each patient may contribute to the improvement—or deterioration—of his own IC. While patients are putting their health on the line, doctors are putting their self-image on the line. The doctor's attitude, therefore, may also fail to be entirely grounded in the here-and-now. The pediatrician who dismissed the mother who asked questions about her children's medications was an extreme example of regression to childish petulance ("You can't play with *my* toys"). More common is the doctor who, when his authority is not immediately deferred to by a patient or SO, or a nurse, masks his insecurity by barking orders or criticizing some unimportant infraction of rules. "Who is in charge here?" is often the underlying question, though the doctor would not deign to voice it.

For whatever the reason, there is a notable discrepancy between what doctors expect of their patients and what the patients actually do. Patients are forever forgetting to take the right amount of medication or perform prescribed exercises. Sometimes their health inertia stems from a natural absentmindedness or laziness, but other times it reflects a hidden resentment of their doctor (or all doctors).

Unconsciously, many a passive-aggressive patient, like Dorothy, would rather frustrate the doctor than get rid of her symptom. Also, people sometimes grow attached to their long-term symptom; it has become one of their characteristics, and friends inquire about its welfare as if it were a member of the family. To give it up would be to feel too much like everyone else. This attitude, like hypochondria, contributes to the apparent paradox that some people exemplify of having a strong will-to-live but a weak will-to-health. On the other side, some people, like Arthur Koestler's wife Cynthia who committed suicide along with him despite her being in good health and some thirty years younger, may exemplify a strong will-to-health but a weak will-to-live.

If a doctor has the bad luck of having a patient with whom he cannot establish a constructive relationship, he has several choices. He can, like Dorothy's doctor, work on himself to try to overcome his antipathy, or he can refer the patient to different kinds of specialists (not an option in a small town), or he can struggle along, finding new drugs to try and making placebo-type recommendations in hope that *something* will galvanize the patient's will-to-health and thus get him off the phone and out of the office.

The underlying pathos in Dorothy's life came from her inability to make friends or enjoy intimacy with anybody. Neither of her parents had modeled this skill for her, and she ended up not truly interested in anyone but herself. Yet to drop her unconscious defenses would have been to assume vulnerability to a degree she dared not risk. Whereas Mary Ellen had indiscriminately reacted to stress by blaming herself, Dorothy indiscriminately blamed other people, which, in turn, made it hard for them to feel friendly toward her.

For most people, friendship is a major way to achieve a wholesome balance (if one can also be friends with one's doctors and nurses, all the better). Samuel Johnson was offering Boswell, in effect, the best of late-twentieth-century health advice when he wrote, "If a man does not make new acquaintances as he advances through life, he will soon find himself left alone. A man, Sir, should keep his friendships in constant repair."

Friendships, in short, need nurturing just as plants do. One form of nurturing is to express interest in the other person, not even fearing, on occasion, to ask a leading question which he is, of course, free not to answer.

Relationships with other people, moreover, do not need to be totally satisfying to improve health on both sides. Marriage is now recognized as a better aid to health and longevity than living alone. Said Leonard Syme, M.D., at an American Heart Association Forum, "What seems to be important is whether or not you're married, not how you feel about it."* The same, he claims, is true of other forms of socializing.

In addition to one-to-one relationships, there is also comembership with other people in small and large groups. A Duke University study concluded that participation in some organization was virtually as significant to maintaining the good health of old people as was their physical and mental, marital and financial condition.

Just as the United States appears to be the country most prone to overguilt, so does it appear to be the one most prone to establishing groups. In these groups, individuals can often ventilate the concerns that are upsetting them, and receive as well as give, useful feedback. As Alexis de Tocqueville noted one hundred fifty years ago in *Democracy in America*: "In no country in the world has the principle of association been more successfully used or applied to a greater multitude of objects than

*A staff-written report, "Perils of Loneliness," *Discover*, March 1982.

in America. Besides the permanent assocations which are established by law . . . a vast number of others are formed and maintained by the agency of private individuals."

Today, the U.S. record for voluntary activity by way of groups is higher than any other country's. And during the past decade there has also been a notable increase in *self-help* organizations. By the early 1980s, fifteen million Americans were taking part in a half million of these. The umbilical cord of most self-help groups is the telephone wire. There is also the predictable regular meeting. One of the earliest, biggest, and most famous of such groups is Alcoholics Anonymous, with its offshoots for spouses and for children (Al-Anon and Al-A-Teen).

For the patient on his own, a difficult first step may be to decide whether he is really sick enough to merit his busy doctor's attention. Dr. Keith Sehnert and Howard Eisenberg, authors of *How to Be Your Own Doctor—Sometimes*, suggest: "You should be able to report . . . temperature, pulse rate . . . respiration rate. . . . You should be able to locate and describe pain—its area (upper right quarter of abdomen), nature (continuous, intermittent, periodic), what makes it better or worse, what symptoms accompany it (nausea, dizziness, fever, etc.), when it began."*

If problems occur in the middle of the night or at other times or places when a doctor is unavailable, one should be aware of home remedies, such as the traditional drinking of liquids, gargling with salt water, applying ice (for sprains, fractures, burns, and cuts) or meat tenderizer (for stings), and use of humidifier (for respiratory congestion).

Today many activated patients have invested in a home encyclopedia and a reference book that describes the effects—and side effects—of prescription and over-the-counter drugs. They also have a blood-pressure cuff, stethoscope, and such items of occasionally used equipment as the home kits for testing pregnancy and diabetes, and the hemocult forms that reveal hidden blood in the stool.†

Dr. Robert Cochran, chief of surgery at Bethesda Naval Hospital, says that if people, especially those over fifty years of age, would use the hemocult forms every six months, the rate of severe colon cancer would be radically reduced.

The activated patient can also learn first-aid techniques and essentials of preventive medicine (see Appendices B, C, D, E, and F). The acquiescent patient, moreover, like the activated one, should learn to ask

---

*Keith Sehnert, M.D., and Howard Eisenberg, *How to Be Your Own Doctor—(Sometimes)* (New York: Putnam, 1981).
†These forms can be mailed to the doctor for evaluation or tested at home by way of a hemocult solution.

for a second opinion when his doctor suggests surgery. Any doctor who objects to having his decision thus reviewed, says Dr. Isadore Rosenfeld, New York cardiologist and author of *Second Opinion*, is paying more attention to his own ego than to the patient's health.

The second opinion in regard to surgery might well be requested *not* from another surgeon but from an internist, lest loyalty to the surgical brotherhood cloud the reviewer's vision.

In the U.S., where surgeons are generally paid a *fee* for the job, far more operations—hysterectomies, for example—are performed than in Britain, where surgeons are on *salary*. This does not mean that American surgeons are necessarily venal; only that, being human, many of them look on their hard-won skill as the best curative agent—as it often is— and tend therefore to be overzealous in recommending it. A common belief is that 25 percent of ailments treated by surgery in America could have been handled with equal success by other means.*

As for tranquilizers, their use in the U.S. reached unprecedented heights in 1980. Some prescriptions were found to result from a doctor's not wanting to spend enough time with his patients to find out the underlying source of their symptoms. Other prescriptions were requested by patients who wanted tangible evidence that their ailment was "real" or that their doctor cared. Because of subsequent health education for the public as well as for doctors, the number of prescriptions for valium and other tranquilizers has dramatically dropped.

Whenever the doctor prescribes a drug new to the patient, the latter should ask about its effect on driving, and about how it acts in combination with any other drugs he is taking, including alcohol, nicotine, caffeine, and large doses of vitamins. Though most people know that alcohol and sleeping pills can be a deadly mixture, few know that mineral oils prevents the absorption of vitamins, or that aspirin may cause stomach bleeding and increase the excretion of vitamin C. Patients may need to be told that tetracycline should not be taken with dairy products and that certain antidepressants should not be taken with such diverse foods as aged cheese, organ meats, mushrooms, pure yeast, chocolate, and chianti. Hosts may soon need to inquire of dinner guests what foods they must avoid, in order to provide a suitable menu!

While activated patients have been turning to support networks of various kinds, so have some doctors. They are joining with lawyers, philosophers, theologians, and social scientists to try to solve some of the agonizing ethical and practical dilemmas created by the progress of med-

---

*A comparison of two neighboring counties in Vermont showed that twice as many hysterectomies were performed in the county with the most ob-gyn surgeons.

ical technology. Examples include what to tell the terminal patient who has asked for the truth but whose family members insist that the diagnosis be kept from him. Others are when to perform amniocentesis, organ transplants, psychosurgery, kidney dialysis, and when to pull the plug on life-sustaining machines if brain death (when no waves register on the electroencephalogram, or EEG) has preceded heart death (when no beats register on the electrocardiogram, or EKG). Should doctors use heroic livesaving equipment on infants born with hideous and irremediable deformities—and give lifesaving medicines such as antibiotics to unresponsive, totally limp retardates whom pneumonia once claimed early in life? To explore such problems and set up criteria by which to judge them, new institutions, such as the Hastings (N.Y.) Institute of Society, Ethics, and the Life Sciences and the Kennedy Institute for Bioethics at Georgetown University, have been established with a combination of private and public funds. Says Dr. Jay I. Meltzer, internist and teacher of medical ethics at Columbia Presbyterian Hospital in New York, "Medicine is less a science than an assessment of risks and benefits."

Precisely because medicine is more potent now than ever before, its implicit values need to be made explicit and reexamined, both by doctors and patients and by legislators and other people interested in improving the quality of health for the individual without bankrupting him or his society.

JUNE: Do patients expect too much from their doctors?

NORMAN: Sometimes they forget we're human; and, I must say, we sometimes forget to remind them.

JUNE: Is medicine too commercialized?

NORMAN: That's a hazard that accompanies specialization. Patients should make sure that their internist is informed about what their various specialists think. Someone besides the patient should be keeping an eye on the *whole* picture.

JUNE: Besides an internist, who could do that?

NORMAN: Some hospitals have a liaison psychiatrist, a professional who can see the problem from the patient's point of view and still be listened to by the specialists.

JUNE: I had a wonderful experience of that kind with a nurse practitioner. She'd had enough special training so that the doctors
had to pay attention to her. At the same time, she didn't pooh-
pooh my perceptions. But a friend of mine in a different hospital finally had to have a temper tantrum and say to his doctor,
"Isn't it too bad that *I* have to accompany *my disease* to your
examining room?"

NORMAN: Fair enough. But don't forget that doctors have cause to lose
their temper too.

JUNE: When?

NORMAN: When patients refuse to "own" their problem and keep blaming
it on someone else. Addictive people, whether alcoholics or
compulsive overeaters like Dorothy, characteristically do that.

JUNE: What other kinds of things make doctors mad?

NORMAN: Repeatedly forgetting their appointment—or arriving very late.

JUNE: But doctors often keep patients waiting—sometimes for hours.

NORMAN: I know, and much of that could—and should—be avoided.
Also, patients try to hide embarrassing facts about themselves.
The doctor really needs to know what's going on in *all* dimensions. He's not expected to make a moral judgment, only
a medical one.

JUNE: But patients are afraid that doctors will talk.

NORMAN: Most doctors are very careful about confidentiality.

JUNE: They gossip with other doctors. If a doctor has to choose between satisfying a colleague's curiosity or being loyal to his
patient, I bet he'll choose his colleague.

NORMAN: But the colleague is also trained to keep his mouth shut.

JUNE: Hmm. What about doctors who have health problems of their
own? I read that some patients are reluctant to go to a psychiatrist who happens to be *physically* handicapped.

NORMAN: It depends on what the handicap is and how well the doctor
has come to grips with it. Often a doctor can be *more* helpful
to a patient in the field of his own previous weakness than a
doctor with no inside experience.

JUNE: So "Physician, heal thyself" can have a ripple effect?

NORMAN: I think so. I also think that doctors have a responsibility to model good health practices.

JUNE: Which ones?

NORMAN: To stay in reasonably good shape and not exhibit too much Type-A behavior.

JUNE: What does that involve?

NORMAN: Always being in a hurry. A form of "time disease." Meyer Friedman who first described the Type-A kind of person called him "a vigilant male beset with internal fury, living in a state of relentless, joyless striving."

JUNE: Good grief, you don't get that way, do you?

NORMAN: Less and less. After all, if we doctors don't practice what we preach, how can we expect our patients to believe us?

XI

New Ways of Well-Being and Exiting

Final Report on Peter

"If a little knowledge is dangerous, where is the man who has so much as to be out of danger?"
—Thomas Henry Huxley

Though Peter liked his new apartment, he badly missed the daily visits from his old card-playing neighbor, Anthony. Still, his daughter Dorothy was living nearby in a furnished room. And on his birthday she had a surprise for him: She had learned gin rummy, his favorite game.

Every day she went over to Peter's and cooked him a hot lunch or supper. He was becoming more arthritic, so she also cleaned for him. He, on the other hand, did not want to become wholly dependent on her. He learned to pick up his newspaper by standing with one foot on each side of it and then bringing his feet together: as the paper humped up, he was able to reach it. With Dorothy's assistance, he had hung two posters. One said, "I'm not retired: I'm recycled"; the other said, "When the going gets tough, the tough get going."

JUNE: Well, Norman, here we are at the last dialogue. What's your view of Peter?

NORMAN: He's a cooney old bird who's learned to roll with the punches. He was right to move away from the apartment with carbon monoxide coming in the window. Still, he missed his old friend. On the other hand, this gap in his life stirred him up to improve his relationship with his daughter—and that was good for *her*, which added momentum to a new mutual wholesome cycle between the two of them.

JUNE: But what will happen to her when he dies?

NORMAN: Hard to say. If she identifies with her mother, she may go into a gradual decline, the way Martha did before she was brought to the hospital with pneumonia. But if Dorothy identifies with her father, she may pull up her socks and find some work and new companionship.

JUNE: She couldn't be a nurse again, could she?

NORMAN: I doubt it. Not with her weight and record and years of being out of touch. The requirements for a nurse today are awesome.

JUNE: Is she still on medication?

NORMAN: A very mild dose. But she's conscientious about taking it.

JUNE: What about Peter?

NORMAN: He, too, is on a mild dose of antidepressant. And Dorothy sees to it that he takes his pill. She also gives him a hard time if he doesn't do his minimal exercises.

JUNE: You mean he has to "use it or lose it"?

NORMAN: Sure. In fact, that theory applies to our social and mental "muscles" as well. The older we get, the more important it is to keep our dimensions in trim. Osteoporosis, for example, is thought to be staved off when people exercise; depression is thought to be staved off when people find a person or group they can feel close to—or do something for. Also, the daily presence of familiar and valued objects can be a boost to morale that helps improve health.

JUNE: But when Peter dies, Dorothy will be all alone.

NORMAN: That's true. And she may unconsciously try to escape her grief by turning paranoid again. Or overeating. Or both. On the other hand, she may become the way Peter was when Martha, following Dorothy's birth, was hospitalized. He was so pleased to be the survivor that his energy increased. Dorothy might be energized to find some other old person who needed a companion like her, with basic nursing skills.

JUNE: And that would keep the old person out of an institution?

NORMAN: It would, and it might also keep Dorothy out of an institution.
           To be adequately healthy, as Dr. René Dubos said, is to be
           able to do what we *want* to do. That gives us two approaches.
           One is to keep up or alter what we are able to do; the other is
           to give up or alter what we want to do. Old age mustn't be
           thought of as a disease; it's a condition, one that all of us, if
           we're *lucky*, will someday attain. And it's one that offers con-
           siderable challenge to each person's IC.

A famous and difficult-to-follow bit of health advice was inscribed
thousands of years ago on the Temple of Apollo at Delphi: "Know thyself."
Self-knowledge involves continuing effort by the IC, perhaps modified
by careful listening to the comments other people make. Sometimes self-
knowledge comes from deliberate self-study, sometimes from the ability
to transcend the self and its situation. Sometimes self-transcendence occurs when the person puts himself in touch with nature, the so-called
below-human; other times it occurs when he tries to put himself in touch
with the purpose of the universe, the beyond-human. Either way, he
harnesses the IC's capacity to mobilize the will or surrender it, to center
the self or expand its reach beyond its grasp.

Although the healing of a localized disorder appears to take place at a
specific area of the body, the *whole* of the person is nonetheless involved.
If Martha, while dying of pneumonia, had needed to have a splinter
removed from her thumb, the excision might never have closed. On the
other hand, New York lawyer Morris Abram was able, through a potent
IC, to mobilize all four of his dimensions and recover from the acute
(myelocytic) leukemia that pervaded his body and that his doctors had
agreed would kill him within a few months. Ten years later he wrote, "I
owe my life first to the advances in chemotherapy; its aggressive use by
physicians, and, of course, my willingness to submit to its risks and
hazards. . . . Also I've had good luck. When I lay in mortal peril during
remission-induction, totally defenseless, I was spared the invasion of
deadly germs. Finally—and I cannot emphasize this enough—I had the
love and support of my family. There was never a day that my wife shared
the conviction of others that I would not survive, and she communicated
in every way . . . her confidence."*

Today a number of ancient health techniques have been rediscovered
and are being used, either alone or in conjunction with modern inven-

*Morris B. Abram, *The Day Is Short* (San Diego: Harcourt Brace Jovanovich, 1982).

tions. For example, meditation is being practiced as a way both to center the self and to find out more *about* the self.*

Meditation's secular manifestation has been named by Dr. Herbert Benson (in his book by that title) *The Relaxation Response*. In many ways it mimics hibernation and provides an alternative to fight or flight. Some serious meditators, for example, need to wrap a blanket around their shoulders because their metabolism drops so sharply. In everyone, at least for a while, blood pressure tends to fall, oxygen intake to be reduced, and brain waves to stretch out into the more peaceful alpha rhythm.

Whether meditation is secular or religious, Doctor Benson says, four elements appear integral to it:
• a repetitive mental device
• a passive attitude
• a decreased muscle tension
• a quiet environment

Some meditators report receiving significant and new signals from their four dimensions. Others report a profound peace of mind. The latter may be connected with an increase in their endorphins. Indeed, for many a regular meditator, serious discomfort may arise if they are forced to skip a day. On the other hand, for certain psychiatric patients (obsessive-compulsives in particular), meditation may be profoundly upsetting, in that too much unconscious material may surface and become over-whelming.

When the mind is centered on a repeated simple sound (a mantra)† or rhythmic process (such as breathing or heartbeat or counting), the usual stream of consciousness is quieted. Thoughts may continue to emerge, but strong emotion is prevented from attaching itself to them. Meditators report a sense of liberation from time, space, even gravity; their limbs feel light, as if their center of gravity were no longer being pulled straight down toward the center of the earth. The consequent relaxation, many claim, is more rejuvenating than sleep. Some evidence is turning up that during meditation more oxygen than usual gets to the

---

*In the sixth century B.C., Hindu scriptures described the technique of attainment of unity with the Universal Spirit by restraining one's breathing and withdrawing sensory attention from the world. In the first century B.C., Jews used a meditative practice of sitting with head between knees, and whispering psalms. In the fourteenth century A.D., Roman Catholics used "the Prayer of the Heart" with similar effect. Rosaries, with repeated prayer or mantra, are still part of Hindu, Moslem, and Roman Catholic ritual.
†Some sounds, such as the Sanscrit "Om" (or the English "one"), when mentally re-peated, elicit slow, flowing brainwaves, while other sounds, such as "Brek," cause rapid, abrupt ones. Aristophanes instinctively gave to his *Frogs* the jarring chorus, "Brekeke-kesh." This was later picked up as a Yale football cheer, used to jangle the team into greater effort.

brain, even though the person's overall consumption of it is reduced. This might explain both the keener thinking that some meditators claim occurs afterward and the finer tuning of the self's inner "radar."

From a religious point of view, the practice of meditation fulfills at least the first part of the Old Testament commandment "Be still—and know that I am God." The IC's essence, moreover, may seem to mingle with that of the cosmos. Says the religiously knowledgeable Paramajamsa Yogananda, "My sense of identity was no longer narrowly confined to a body but embraced the circumambient atoms. People on distant streets seemed to be moving over my own remote periphery. . . . My ordinary frontal vision was now changed to a vast spherical sight. . . . An oceanic joy broke upon calm endless shores of my soul."*

Some people report that their experience of meditation provides an internal bomb shelter of sorts. As one meditator said, "It enables you to rise above even nuclear war, because the spirit which is our essence, and to which we open ourselves in meditation, cannot be destroyed."

Meditation may also provide an expansion of the imaginative power to grasp the interdependence of all life on Earth, including our own. This connection was dramatized in 1968 when astronauts returned with a photo of Planet Earth, blue and white, vulnerable and alone, in the vast blackness of space. Twenty years before, British astrophysicist Fred Hoyle had predicted, "Once a photograph of the earth . . . is available . . . once the sheer isolation . . . becomes plain, a new idea as powerful as any in history will be let loose."

This powerful idea is working its ferment on both sides of the Iron Curtain and may yet succeed in protecting the health of all human beings now and in the future—not to mention the previous legacy of art, literature, science, and history—by preventing nuclear war from being used as any kind of a solution. †

Related to secular meditation is biofeedback, a typically American invention that operates at the interface between technology and the individual. Today some Americans of every age and station are attaching sensors to their skin to measure changes registered by machines that beep or go silent, light up or turn dim, depending on whether the person's meditative technique is resulting in relaxing his forehead, dropping his blood pressure, slowing his heart, increasing the alpha waves of his brain

---

*Paramajamsa Yogananda, The Autobiography of a Yogi (Los Angeles: Self Realization Fellowship, 1971).
†Dr. Eugene I. Chasov, deputy minister of health in the U.S.S.R., and personal physician to several recent chairmen of the Soviet Union, was one of the first important Russian Communist Party members to make clear to his countrymen the impossibility of either side winning a major nuclear exchange.

or the temperature of either or both his hands. To find oneself capable of controlling internal forces that, until recently, were thought to be beyond reach by anyone other than a highly trained Eastern mystic may itself provide elation, which, in turn, may interrupt an unwanted cycle.

Neal E. Miller, M.D., the grandfather of biofeedback, has helped patients thus to obtain relief from chronic pain and asthmatic breathing, hypertension (partly in order to prevent stroke), and some paralysis (following stroke).

Another introspective technique is visualization. Dr. O. Carl Simonton, a radiation oncologist in Fort Worth, Texas, suggests that during and after surgery, radiation, and chemotherapy, cancer patients enter a meditative state and then picture in living color their white cells, or other aspect of their immune system, destroying whatever helpless cancer cells may remain.* One of his students pictures the white cells as white polar bears, which gobble up black grapefruit-size suspicious-looking cells, as twice a day he gradually moves his mental eye internally from the top of his head to the soles of his feet.

In another form of visualization, Dr. Harold Wise, of Montefiore Hospital in the Bronx, tells patients to picture their cancer cells as immature "baby" cells that need to be programmed by the patient in order to be useful, rather than dangerous, to him.

Not everyone wishes to meditate, let alone practice biofeedback or visualization. But everyone may need, at one time or another, to mobilize his IC to bring the maturity levels of the four dimensions into alignment.

Yet in the United States today, this is often not easy, particularly for the young. In the dimension of *body*, for example, better nutrition and other factors have lowered the average age of puberty by almost two years since the turn of the century. In the realm of *mind*, this shortening of childhood has meant for many youngsters a lack of opportunity to work through the profound emotions naturally connected with parents and other archetypal figures. Children, it seems, need to feel and act like children for a certain number of years in order to facilitate their IC growth. Yet today's *environments* are such that children at a tender age are repeatedly exposed through the media to explicit violence and sex. (Youngsters *not* limited in their TV viewing are found to picture the world as a more threatening and violent place than are youngsters who see only age-

---

*In *Advances*, Summer 1984, Martin L. Rossman, M.D., a board member of the Institute for the Advancement of Health, writes, "Carl Simonton and Stephanie Mathews Simonton . . . have reported . . . that people with advanced cancers who involve themselves in a program of visualization . . . significantly extend their lives when compared to the statistical prognoses of cancer patients who do not. . . . This research deserves the most careful efforts at well-designed, properly controlled replication."

appropriate programs.) As for *relationships with people*, American children's chances of growing up together with both natural parents are now less than fifty-fifty.

Small wonder that people keep complaining of how hard it is to get their act (or IC) together. An imbalance in the relative maturity of their four dimensions may also add to difficulty in navigating the transitions between the predictable life stages—what Gail Sheehy, in her book by that title, called *passages*. Achieving public recognition of their private passage to a new form of commitment may be the motive behind so many modern couples' insistence on the rite of an old-fashioned wedding, complete with white dress and cake, even if, in contemporary fashion, the couple had been living together for years.

For the *nation* to get its health act together involves extremely difficult decisions. How should we allot which funds to which private and public agencies under which conditions? Less obvious, but also important, is the need to protect individual privacy from the storage of health data already going on. Many an overly inquisitive government or industry official, political opponent or personal enemy, has been startled by the computer response "Not allowed to reveal unless inquirer has special key."

In the short run, sophisticated medical technology increases the expense of health care, with some pills costing more than a dollar apiece, and some diagnostic machinery costing more than one hundred thousand dollars a year just to run, not to mention the more-than-one-million-dollars needed to buy it. Yet in the long run, medical technology may end up saving not only millions of lives but billions of dollars.

In the past, many drugs were discovered by serendipity: as a by-product of the search for something else. One such discovery occurred in 1928 when bacteriologist Alexander Fleming noticed a strange mold cluttering his laboratory dishes of asperfillis and penicillium. Curiosity led him to investigate further: The result of this chance observation was penicillin. Still, as Pasteur observed, "Chance favors the prepared mind." Today, in contrast, many drugs are deliberately being designed to augment natural substances produced in the human body. Through recombinant DNA, for example, a form of insulin similar to that produced by the human pancreas is being "grown" in rapidly reproducing laboratory bacteria. Such minifactories have also been established to produce interferon, a naturally occurring antiviral agent that also reduces some tumors. And the search is on for chemicals that will bestir the body to increase its own supply of interferon and other materials used by the immune system.

In addition to antiviral agents, there are antibacterial ones, such as the newly discovered lymphotoxin and tumor necrosis factor. Produced by the human body in infinitessimal quantities, their presence had previously been surmised because tumors shrank or even disappeared in some cancer patients who developed severe bacterial infections.

In experiments with animals, lymphotoxin and tumor necrosis factor have successfully killed off tumor cells together with unwanted bacteria. In the laboratory, these products can now be made in unlimited quantities. The hope, according to Jan Vicek, M.D., a microbiologist at New York University Medical School, is that in humans these or similar agents can combat tumor cells without harming normal cells, as current radiation and chemotherapy tend to do. *

In still another development, fast-growing bone-marrow cancer (myeloma) cells, combined with human spleen cells, have produced an artificial cell (hybridoma) that is expected to concoct chemicals that may prevent hepatitis, malaria, even cancer. And humulin, a new form of insulin thus produced, is on the market. Longer-term possibilities include organ cloning for old people through removal and freezing of organ cells during their youth. Already, a snippet of a burn patient's skin can be rapidly grown in the laboratory into sizable sheets that the patient's body will not reject.

Improvements in *cure* for a relatively few people are being rivaled in dramatic impact by improvements in *prevention* of ailments for the millions. During the past ten years, for example, some five thousand corporations have instituted employee health-assistance programs. Originally started in order to treat alcoholism and drug abuse, these programs have broadened to include such preventive measures as teaching good nutrition, encouraging exercise, discouraging smoking, and instituting screening for hypertension and cancer. More than five hundred companies have set up "wellness plans," often with AFL-CIO encouragement. New York Telephone Company doctors, for example, claim a 90 percent success rate in treating employee hypertension, an important step in prevention of heart disease and stroke.

Some companies reward employees who take action to stay well. The Hospital Corporation of America, for instance, pays employees by the mile to swim or jog. Dow Chemical (Texas division) pays cash to employees who give up smoking.

Over the years, the most efficient way to reduce health costs is through education. A three-year "Feelin' Good" program in Jackson County, Michigan, has increased the health know-how of twenty-four thousand schoolchildren and significantly decreased their body fat, blood choles-

*Associated Press, "Rare Anticancer Agents Made in Laboratories," *New York Times*, January 1 1985.

terol, and blood pressure. Children are fascinated by their bodies, adolescents by their emotions. At the college level, academic credit is given for the study of both the capacities and limitations of physiology and psychology. At Barnard College, for example, the catalog states, "*Health and Society* is . . . a program to [establish] causes in the health sciences, to identify limits of scientific knowledge . . . and develop decision-making skills under conditions of scientific uncertainty."

The sciences, in short, have crested the foothills only to glimpse the challenging snow-capped mountains ahead.

The two most dramatic individual *passages*—namely, birth and death—are often handled in ways that combine the best of old common sense and new technology. Modern birthing techniques involve, as before general anesthesia, a conscious mother with a significant other in attendance. Novel is the way that, through childbirth training (or perhaps a local anesthetic), the mother is neither in unbearable pain nor suffering the fearful anticipation of pain that, in a vicious cycle, formerly exacerbated suffering. Her IC feels the stronger for maintaining some control. And her sense of control, in benign cycle, is strengthened by encouragement from her significant other (or doctor or midwife) when she succeeds in riding a wave of pain rather than being tumbled by it.

In many modern birthing clinics, her room is quiet and the light soft. She can relax, even drop off, between contractions. Many women report a wondrous feeling of being in tune with the fundamental purpose of the universe: the continuance of life. Others rejoice in being able to trust the miraculous powers of their own body. Still others feel the closeness of "the everlasting arms." Such women come through the experience with not only a new baby but also a newly strengthened IC.*

The mother's self-confidence may provide her with extra impetus to care well for the baby, and may communicate itself in soothing ways to the baby, who then may behave in a cooperative manner. Thus a mutually reinforcing and wholesome cycle may be established for *both* generations.

In some quarters, the final rite of passage is viewed as the IC's ultimate challenge, and preparation for dying is carefully thought out by the patient, together perhaps with close family members, friends, and doctor. "The Living Will" (Appendix H) leaves clear instructions about not using machines to keep the patient going after meaningful life has become an impossibility. The organ-donor card offers the dying person a sense of continuity as needed body parts, such as corneas or even a heart, may offer new life to another person.

---

*Not every woman is equipped for natural childbirth, nor is every mate. Guilt, therefore, should not be attributed or felt when other methods are chosen.

Some terminal patients hasten their end through an overdose of sleeping pills in order to avoid excruciating pain of body, collapse of mind, or even financial disaster for the family. Someday the old Eskimo practice may be more widely adopted: of offering honor to the family whose Old One, at the appropriate time, chooses to walk out into the snow. On the other hand, for the family to *force* her—or him—into such a step would still be murder.

Many people try to help their dying person leave no unfinished emotional business between self and family members. Sometimes family and friends make a concerted effort to meet with the patient, well *ahead of* the time for the funeral. New York internists Harold Wise and Charles Goodrich make a practice of encouraging such bedside reunions. Or if a significant other cannot make the necessary long trip, he is asked to stop and send thoughts or prayers toward the patient at the exact time when the others are foregathering. Just as the "evil eye" can injure, so can hopeful vibrations heal—or at least soothe or provide a lift. Hubert Humphrey, while hospitalized for the bladder cancer that ultimately claimed his life, reported in 1978 that for him it was "a spiritual experience" to receive word that congregations in churches and synagogues all over the world were praying for him (fifty thousand letters also were received): "I want to tell you, my friend, I could feel it, actually feel it. It came to me with a great surge of healing. I could feel it in my body, the warmth, the friendship, the prayers. It was really like a healing balm. I know it sounds almost irrational. I can't explain it, but I know something was happening to me and I was getting strength from it."

Family members too, may derive strength from reunion with the dying person, especially if forgiveness can be shared and ancient differences relegated to the trash heap of irrelevance. When no overguilt remains between the dying person and those who deeply care, death may be peaceful and the legacy a wholesome one.

Dr. Harold Wise tells of a young man who asked his first cousin, whom he had not seen since their mutual grandmother's death the previous year, "Do you still talk to Grandma?"

"All the time! Do you?"

"Oh sure, and what's more, she answers back."

For religious people, their faith may offer solace against the Grim Reaper. Some look forward to rejoining loved ones already dead. Some consider it liberation to cast off "this old pillowcase," as Hindus, Buddhists, or Sikhs may refer to the body. At the same time, nonreligious people may be comforted by the sense that their death fits into a preordained wider system, since, throughout nature, death and decay—"We are all biodegradable"—are essential prelude to the emergence of new life.

Though the purpose of modern medicine is to prolong living, a by-product has been to prolong dying. Yet much of the terminal agony so shattering to the IC is now being ameliorated through the hospice movement. Founded at Saint Christopher's in London by Dr. Cecily Saunders, this combination of love-bringing people and pain-banishing drugs administered *before* the pain has time to arise enables the patient's IC to retain its characteristic pattern to the end.

Instrumental in bringing the hospice movement to the United States were writers Victor and Rosemary Zorza.* Their daughter Jane, an intelligent, temperamental young woman of twenty-five, dying in anguish from melanoma, was admitted to a hospice near Oxford, England. After her pain was brought under control, her parents observed that "her heightened sensitivity made it possible to perceive her own feelings and those of others in a way she had never done before."

They quote her as saying, "I feel I have learned quite a lot that maybe I knew intellectually before, but not emotionally. . . . I appreciate things (the beautiful ones, anyway) and people (the nice ones) much more."

Though the quantity of Jane's life was cruelly abbreviated, its quality was poignantly expanded.

For many older people, loss of mental faculties and consequent damage to their IC is far worse than loss of life. Fortunately, research on Alzheimer's and Parkinson's diseases, as well as similar forms of localized brain malfunction, is now being funded, and many young doctors are heading into this promising field. In Sweden, for example, implants of cells that produce dopamine have been experimentally placed in brains of patients with Parkinson's disease.

In the United States, it was to the free individual that the founding fathers delegated "the pursuit of happiness." Today it is to the free and informed individual that science is delegating the pursuit of health. Individuals in a democracy are also freer than those in a dictatorship to decide together how to apply their individual and small-group IC strengths to correct hazards from the environments. †

Among the crucial self-help groups are those that combine devotion to their nation with refusal to stay quiet when it defines its self-interest too narrowly. What they hope to prevent is some other country's feeling

*Victor and Rosemary Zorza, A Way to Die (New York: Knopf, 1980).
†An important area of such action, according to the National Academy of Sciences, is collecting valid data about the sixty-five thousand chemicals on the American market. According to the Academy's 1984 study, "Of tens of thousands of commercially important chemicals, only a few have been subjected to extensive toxicity testing."

so cornered by theirs that in desperation it launches a nuclear war. Dr. Jonas Salk, author of *Millennium*, indirectly refers to this kind of IC power when he says that although, in the course of evolution, many more species have become extinct than have survived, the human species can survive if it develops the kind of "wisdom . . . for which a balanced creative center is required."

"A balanced creative center" at the individual level is the product not of mind alone but of all four dimensions working together under IC direction. At the group level, such a balanced creative center is the product not of one leader alone but of many people's IC's working together in cooperative fashion. (Even in a dictatorship, the leader is dependent on the opinions of those people close to him.) Already, many people with sufficient courage to care and act are striving in self-correcting and healing concert to improve the well-being of this fragile planet and its present and future inhabitants.

For millennia, people have been given the moral reasons for love, and the spiritual reasons as well.

Today we are given the medical reasons for love.

This love incorporates the kind we have traditionally been asked to feel for neighbor and self. But today science has obliterated the total distinction between these two individuals, just as earlier it had wiped out the total distinction between any single individual's body and mind. As a result, the person considered by modern medicine to be glowingly alive is the one whose self-interest is not encapsulated but has broadened and deepened to embrace the well-being of those individuals and groups, environments and ideals to which he is joined in intimate connection.

Appendices

Common-Sense Rules of Diet

(culled from the syndicated newspaper columns by pioneer nutritionist Jean Mayer, M.D., now president of Tufts University)

1. Avoid excess salt and sugar.

2. Keep low one's consumption of red meat, primarily beef and lamb, and substitute fish and poultry, legumes and grains, nuts and seeds.

3. Substitute low-fat milk for whole milk, low-fat cheese for high-fat cheese.

4. Substitute polyunsaturated margarine and vegetable oils for butter, lard, and bacon fat.

5. Eat plenty of fruits, and green and leafy, as well as yellow, vegetables, raw and cooked.

The Social Readjustment Rating Scale

(compiled by Drs. T. H. Holmes and R. H. Rahe)

EVENTS	SCALE OF IMPACT
Death of spouse	100
Divorce	73
Marital separation	65
Jail term	63
Death of close family member	63
Personal injury or illness	53
Marriage	50
Fired at work	47
Marital reconciliation	45
Retirement	45
Change in health of family member	44
Pregnancy	40
Sex difficulties	39
Addition of new family member	39
Business readjustment	39
Change in financial state	38
Death of close friend	37
Change to different line of work	36
Change in number of arguments with spouse	35
Mortgage over $10,000	31
Foreclosure of mortgage or loan	30
Change in responsibilities at work	29
Son or daughter leaving home	29
Trouble with in-laws	29
Outstanding personal achievement	28
Spouse begins or stops work	26
Begin or end school	26
Change in living conditions	25
Revision of personal habits	24

Trouble with boss	23
Change in work hours or conditions	20
Change in residence	20
Change in schools	20
Change in recreation	19
Change in church activities	19
Change in social activities	18
Mortgage or loan less than $10,000	17
Change in sleeping habits	16
Change in number of family get-togethers	15
Change in eating habits	15
Vacation	13
Christmas	12
Minor violations of the law	11

(Note that twenty-two of the forty-three events are connected with *relationships with people.*)

The Fleeting Symptoms That May Herald a Stroke

- Numbness or weakness in a limb or facial muscle.
- Difficulty in speaking or swallowing.
- Blurry or double vision.
- Deafness or ringing in the ear(s).
- Fainting, dizziness, or mild loss of balance.
- Sudden unusual headache.
- Abrupt and unusual irritability, suspiciousness, or forgetfulness.

These TIA's (Transient Ischemic Attacks) should be immediately reported to the doctor. In the interim before she or he calls back, an aspirin (which acts as a mild anticlotting agent) might be taken.

General Health Regimen

Recommended by Dr. Norman Tamarkin
(who does not always follow it)

1. Get seven or eight hours of sleep a night.

2. Eat breakfast, especially high-fiber foods and fruits.

3. Keep weight normal in relation to height.

4. Don't smoke.

5. Exercise on a regular basis.

6. Drink only in moderation (a glass or two of wine or beer per day, and spirits only occasionally).

7. Burn the candle at only one end (i.e., if you work too hard, then don't play too hard, or if you play too hard, then don't work too hard; alternate periods of overexertion with periods of rest, and periods of laziness with periods of self-galvanizing).

Signals of Depression

(listed by Dr. John Kane, director of Long Island Jewish–Hillside Medical Center's Depression Clinic, Hillside, New York)

If, for no evident reason, more than six of the following symptoms develop, the person should check with a doctor in regard to depression:

1. Feelings of sadness, hopelessness ("I will never improve").

2. Loss of "pleasure capacity," the ability to enjoy.

3. Loss of usual interest in sex.

4. Loss of appetite (or overeating).

5. Insomnia (or sleeping too much).

6. Anxious or restless behavior (or apathy).

7. Difficulty in concentration, memory, decision-making.

8. Becoming unduly upset by small things.

9. Feelings of worthlessness ("I'm no good").

10. Withdrawal from friends and relatives.

Eight Signals That May Indicate Cancer

1. Uncharacteristic constipation (or perhaps diarrhea), gas pains, severe indigestion, loss of appetite, rectal bleeding.

2. In the mouth, a painless sore or a raised, irregular warty area; a lump or thickening of the cheek, gum, or tongue.

3. In the throat, difficulty in swallowing, persistent hoarseness; a "lump in the throat," soreness in the neck.

4. On the skin, a sore that does not heal, a dry scaly patch, a pimple that persists, an inflamed area with a crusting center, or a pale, waxy, pearly nodule; most serious and demanding *immediate* attention, a dark brown or black molelike growth that becomes larger, more irregular in shape, or eventually ulcerates and bleeds.

5. In the lungs, a cough that persists (heavy smokers should have frequent lung examinations).

6. For men: any continuing urinary difficulty, lower back, pelvic or, upper-thigh pain, or blood in the urine (the latter is also a danger signal for women).

7. For women: unusual bleeding or discharge from the vagina (all women should have a Pap smear performed once a year and practice breast self-examination once a month or more frequently); any lump or thickening or unusual puckering of the skin of the breast; unusual nipple discharge.

8. In the brain, unremitting headaches, loss of coordination, abrupt changes in personality.

Facts You Should Have for the Emergency Room

Any day—or night—you could become one of the millions who are rushed to American hospitals every month for emergency treatment. An idle warning? American Hospital Association figures show that more than 82.8 million emergency cases were handled in 1978 alone. That's more than one-third of our total population. And a trip to the hospital is usually the sort of thing that happens just when you least expect it.

So what can you do about it? Be prepared, wherever you are, with the answers hospital personnel need to speed your case—answers that, even if you don't arrive unconcious or alone, friends and loved ones would be hard-pressed to provide. In short, carry with you at all times certain basic information that can be of vital importance when every minute counts. Our research indicates you should have:

1. Your name, address, phone number, physical description, and identifying marks (even a passport-type photo), and information on your doctor and others to notify in the event of an emergency.

2. Your occupation and your employer's name, address, and phone number; your social-security number, Medicare and Medicaid numbers if you have them; the name and address of a "Responsible Party," and information on any hospitalization insurance you have.

3. A quick-check list giving your blood type, allergies and/or drug sensitivities; immunizations (including the date of your last tetanus booster); notice if you have a history of such problems as heart trouble, diabetes or epilepsy; and a notation of any organs removed or any implants.

4. Brief details on your current medication (including dosage and precise identification of drugs); comments on significant medical problems; your surgical history (including dates and physicians); and information on prior hospital admissions.

This material should be clearly identified, organized as precisely as possible, and always available. The trouble you take in preparing it will be more than compensated by the knowledge that it might well be of key importance in speeding your admission, diagnosis, treatment, and recovery.

173

Tips for Keeping Off Weight When Giving Up Smoking

The American Heart Association, aware that many smokers, especially women, fear that they will gain weight if they give up smoking, has issued several tips about weight control. Among them are:

- Choose foods that keep your hands busy, such as unshelled nuts.
- Chew sugarless gum.
- Use artificially sweetened mints, letting the candy melt slowly.
- For snacks, keep a supply of cut raw vegetables and unbuttered popcorn.
- Keep high-calorie foods out of the house if possible, and certainly out of sight.
- Have someone else put away the leftovers.
- Slow down your eating by cutting food into smaller pieces, putting the fork down between bites, sipping water.
- Temporarily avoid alcohol, which adds calories and diminishes willpower.
- Choose fruit or low-fat milk from vending machines.
- Exercise.
- Don't get discouraged. Most women who gain weight after giving up smoking only put on five or ten pounds, and even this weight is likely to disappear over the course of a year. To equal the health risks associated with cigarette smoking, you would have to gain one hundred pounds!

LIVING WILL DECLARATION

To My Family, Doctors, and All Those Concerned with My Care

I, _____ , being of sound mind, make this statement as a directive to be followed if for any reason I become unable to participate in decisions regarding my medical care.

I direct that life-sustaining procedures should be withheld or withdrawn if I have an illness, disease or injury, or experience extreme mental deterioration, such that there is no reasonable expectation of recovering or regaining a meaningful quality of life.

These life-sustaining procedures that may be withheld or withdrawn include, but are not limited to:

SURGERY   ANTIBIOTICS   CARDIAC RESUSCITATION
RESPIRATORY SUPPORT   ARTIFICIALLY ADMINISTERED FEEDING AND FLUIDS

I further direct that treatment be limited to comfort measures only, even if they shorten my life.

You may delete any provision above by drawing a line through it and adding your initials.

Other personal instructions:

These directions express my legal right to refuse treatment. Therefore, I expect my family, doctors, and all those concerned with my care to regard themselves as legally and morally bound to act in accord with my wishes, and in so doing to be free from any liability for having followed my directions.

Signed _____ Date _____

Witness _____ Witness _____

PROXY DESIGNATION CLAUSE

If you wish, you may use this section to designate someone to make treatment decisions if you are unable to do so. Your Living Will Declaration will be in effect even if you have not designated a proxy.

I authorize the following person to implement my Living Will Declaration by accepting, refusing and/or making decisions about treatment and hospitalization:

Name _____

Address _____

If the person I have named above is unable to act on my behalf, I authorize the following person to do so:

Name _____

Address _____

I have discussed my wishes with these persons and trust their judgment on my behalf.

Signed _____ Date _____

Witness _____ Witness _____

Courtesy of Society for the Right to Die, 250 West 57 Street, New York, NY 10107.

Index